Scenes of action in a modern hospital —dramatic and personal, earthy and warmly human—reveal the real problems of patients and doctors, seen from the inside.

HOSPITAL CHAPLAIN
by Kenneth R. Mitchell

The world of the hospital is one most of us know only as patients—or as visitors with an "outsider's" point of view. This revealing look into the heart of hospital life shows the drama we suspect, but seldom see, hidden behind thick walls.

Here are human issues and emotional crises that arise daily in that highly charged place—where so many decisions must be made that have nothing to do with drugs or surgery. The names are changed to protect privacy, but the events are real. The patients, physicians, surgeons, and chaplains in these stories, and many of the actual conversations, are taken directly from the author's experiences.

Kenneth Mitchell discusses the work, both routine and unusual, that a chaplain does. He begins by relating the crises he encounters in an "average" day, giving an in-depth view of people and problems. The rest of the book is organized around the crucial situations that his work involves: birth, surgery, work with children, with students, with hospital staff, with the dying, and with all kinds of human beings of different faiths, different backgrounds, different needs. Few areas of life are untouched.

(Continued on back flap)

HOSPITAL CHAPLAIN

Books by KENNETH R. MITCHELL
Published by THE WESTMINSTER PRESS

*Psychological and Theological Relationships
in the Multiple Staff Ministry*
Hospital Chaplain

HOSPITAL CHAPLAIN

by Kenneth R. Mitchell

THE WESTMINSTER PRESS
Philadelphia

Grateful acknowledgment is made to Little, Brown and Company for permission to reprint the poem "Notes for the Chart in 306." Copyright © 1966 by Ogden Nash. This poem originally appeared in *The New Yorker*.

PUBLISHED BY THE WESTMINSTER PRESS ®
PHILADELPHIA, PENNSYLVANIA

PRINTED IN THE UNITED STATES OF AMERICA

Library of Congress Cataloging in Publication Data

Mitchell, Kenneth R
  Hospital chaplain.

  1. Chaplains, Hospital. I. Title.
BV4335.M58   253.5   72-76438
ISBN 0-664-20946-7

FOR JUDY

—WHO PAID THE PRICE WITH ME
—AND ALL TOO OFTEN FOR ME

CONTENTS

Foreword   9

I. A Chaplain   11

II. A Day   18

III. Birth   31

IV. Children   41

V. Medicine   50

VI. Surgery   60

VII. Psychiatry   73

VIII. Death   87

IX. Students   97

X. Behind the Stairs   110

XI. Patienthood   118

FOREWORD

IN WRITING THIS BOOK, I have intended to do three things.

First, I wanted to share my experiences as a hospital chaplain. The world of the hospital is a world most of us know as patients. Church people, both laymen and pastors, know the hospital as a place where they visit others. I knew the hospital as a place where I lived, struggled, rejoiced, and wept. That very real experience has stayed with me.

Second, I wanted to try to say what is at stake in hospital life. Issues arise every day and are handled on the run. Ethical decisions have to be made. Everybody who works in a hospital has to use skills that have little to do with drugs and surgical tools. Those skills, those decisions, and those issues are to me the heart of medical care.

Third, I wanted to say something to pastors who *can* and who *must* do the same kind of work, though perhaps not with the same intensity. The kind of care a chaplain extends is pastoral care, and it is done daily by many parish pastors.

You may wonder if Samuel Perkins is Kenneth Mitchell, or if Midbank University Hospital is Vanderbilt University Hospital, where I served as chaplain. The answer is yes—and no. For the most part Sam Perkins' experiences are mine, but a few of the incidents in the book happened not to me but to my students and colleagues. Sam Perkins represents me, but he also represents others. In the same way, Midbank University

Hospital is Vanderbilt Hospital, and it isn't. It's Barnes Hospital in Saint Louis, Billings Hospital in Chicago, and several other hospitals in other places. Anything that happens in this book could have happened, and probably did, in those other hospitals.

But I am dealing in this book with real things that happened to real patients, real physicians and surgeons, and real chaplains. To convey that reality, and to protect it, I have done two things.

I have changed names, promoted and demoted doctors in and out of their real hospital positions, altered times, ages, cultural backgrounds, and other identifying marks. My hope is that I have protected the confidentiality so often entrusted to me by students and patients. No one in the book appears *exactly* as he or she is in real life. What I have not changed are the feelings, thoughts, and actions of human beings.

The other thing I have done is this: I have preserved many conversations exactly as they took place. The hospital is a highly emotional place, and under the pressure of feelings, people use language that is casual, loaded with feelings, and sometimes crude. What we often hear in a hospital is language that has been laundered and perhaps sterilized. Behind the careful, official talk the patient hears is another kind of talk: angry, often coarse and even offensive, but always human. I am unwilling to delete that humanity for the sake of avoiding offense. In some cases, as in the chapter on childbirth, the humanity so vigorously expressed is the key to understanding what is going on.

I could, I know, make a list of all the physicians, surgeons, pastors, and other colleagues who shared in these ministries, and I could and probably should say "Thank you" to all of them. But as I look back, I find that my most deeply felt gratitude goes to my wife, who felt the pain and the struggle, often even when I was unable to share it fully—and to the patients. And to the patients.

K.R.M.

I

A CHAPLAIN

AT THREE THIRTY A.M. the halls were hushed. I stood for a moment at the intersection of D Hall and T Hall, still shaking off sleep. Off to the right, along D Hall, Sue Puckett, the night charge nurse on Pediatrics, sat in her bright alcove, scribbling. If I went down there, Sue would utter the classic nurse's complaint about nursing being all paper work and little patient care. I looked up and down the bright halls.

A place that's dark and quiet is difficult if you have a few fears to cope with. But a place that's absolutely silent but brightly lighted is positively eerie.

The Pediatrics Conference Room, T-330, was just ahead. That was where Abe Chusid was waiting for me, perhaps with someone in trouble, perhaps alone. I went in.

"Hi, Abe."

"Hello, Sam. Glad you could come. This couple's eighteen-month-old child just died, and we don't know why. Will you talk to them?"

"Sure. What should I know?"

"Mostly that they've been married eight years, and this was their only child. They'd tried like hell to get pregnant, and finally saw Chet Norris; he got them going. This kid was the center of their lives. Tell you more later, after you've seen them. I've got a post permission." (A slip permitting the hospital's pathologists to conduct a postmortem examination.)

"O.K. I'll see them now. Where are they?"

"Right next door. Bill and Elaine Watt."

Abe Chusid, a pediatrician in private practice and a member of the teaching staff in the Pediatrics Department, had called me at home. Surprising how polite and formal he was over the phone.

"Is Chaplain Perkins there?"

I recognized his voice, but I was formal too.

"This is he."

"Sam. Abe Chusid. I've got a tough one here at the hospital. Can you come down?"

"Twenty minutes, Abe. O.K.?"

"O.K. I'll meet you in the peds conference room." (Peds, pronounced "peeds"—pediatrics.)

I knew Abe Chusid well. He was our own choice to care for our children. In fact, Janet had taken our own toddler to Abe's office that afternoon for her DPT. (A combined injection to protect children against *D*iphtheria, *P*ertussis [whooping cough], and *T*etanus.) Over coffee, Abe and I had often talked about dealing with the parents of dying children: what you tell them, when you tell them, how you tell them. Now all the coffee-shop conferences came back. All the certainties of three in the afternoon faded, replaced by the uncertainties of three in the morning.

"Mr. and Mrs. Watt? I'm Chaplain Perkins."

"Thank you for coming." (*Lord, how we stick to the polite formulas! Sometimes they're all we have.*)

Their faces were completely blank. When we say someone is grief-stricken we often think of twisted, tortured faces. But this is more common. The face of grief is, at first, a face wiped clean of all expression. Blank. Empty.

"Would you like to tell me what happened?"

"Well, there's nothing to tell. We'd had a party that lasted until after midnight. We stayed up to do the dishes, and finished about one thirty. I went in to check on Ricky while Bill put the cat out. Ricky wasn't breathing. I picked him up, and he was limp. I knew he was dead. Bill called Dr. Chusid, and he met us here at the hospital."

Her voice was as blank as her face.

Bill spoke in the same empty voice. "You're the chaplain of the hospital?"

"Yes."

"We aren't religious people. Elaine was Evangelical and Reformed, and I was Jewish. When we got married, we discovered we weren't really churchy people, so we didn't go anywhere. But it's nice of you to come."

"Perhaps you're wondering about talking to a chaplain?"

"Dr. Chusid said you'd understand how we feel. Do you?"

"I wonder if you might not feel just about as empty as you look."

(*Should I help them cry? They'll need to cry, but can they?*)

"Maybe empty is the word. We don't even know what's happened. Did we do the right thing in signing that autopsy thing, Bill?"

"I think so. We want to know what happened, don't we? Isn't that right, Chaplain . . . —uh—"

"Perkins. Sam Perkins. Would you feel better, do you think, if you knew what had happened to Ricky?"

"Oh, I want to know. He was just fine this afternoon, playing outside. And now he's . . ."

Unable to finish her sentence, Elaine Watt was finally able to cry. Sobbing, she leaned on her husband, who, machine-like, put an arm around her. He looked at me as if to ask if it was all right to comfort his wife.

"Mr. Watt, maybe you'd rather sit together on this couch."

"Thank you, you're very kind."

(*For what? For calling your attention to a couch where you can let your body touch your wife's?*)

Still holding her, he looked at me again, obviously puzzled.

"Chaplain, may I ask you a question?"

"Sure."

"What do we do about a funeral?"

"Well, what puzzles you about that?"

"Well, as I said, we aren't church people. We were starting to talk about going together to the Unitarian Church, but we hadn't done anything about it. I guess what I'm afraid of is one of those god-awful funeral home services, so pompous and all. I couldn't stand that."

Elaine Watt sat up, wiped her tears, became alert.

"Me neither. This is hell, but this isn't what I want to remember. Could we have something, do something, that would be all happy, like Ricky was?"

"You want your good feelings about Ricky to be there in the funeral service."

"Yes, oh, yes."

"Maybe the funeral might be something that would have in it *all* your feelings."

"What do you mean, Chaplain?"

"It seems to me that you do have loads of happy feelings about Ricky's life with you. But you also have hurt feelings and angry feelings, don't you?"

"God, yes! You mean the funeral should express those too?"

"That depends on what you think a funeral should be for."

By now it was obvious that, for now, talking about the funeral was the way the Watts were going to keep their feelings under control. Elaine could let her pain out; I wasn't so sure about Bill.

During the next year, I would see Bill and Elaine Watt several more times.

Bill chopped off the end of his finger with an ax, had the wound dressed in the Emergency Room, and "casually" came by the Chaplain's Office on his way out.

Elaine came in for minor surgery and called from her bedside.

Finally, almost a year to the day after Ricky's death, I walked with Bill Watt up and down the hall outside the Delivery Room while Chet Norris helped Elaine deliver a new child.

What about Ricky's funeral? It was held in the tiny hospital chapel. Bill and Elaine Watt invited friends to come. We expressed their sorrow, their pain, and their anger. We also celebrated their joy in having had Ricky. In the back by the door, with his long white hospital coat, stood Dr. Abe Chusid.

Chaplain.

What does the word mean?

To word lovers, it's a word with an interesting history. Saint Martin, in Christian legend, divided his cloak with a beggar. (The beggar, one version says, was Christ returned to earth.) The small cloak that the saint had left—in Latin, *cappella*— became a famous relic, guarded by a group of priests calling themselves *cappellani*. After a while, cappellani was the name used for clergymen who were not attached to a church.

To dictionary makers, a chaplain is a clergyman who offers a religious ministry to a special group: a military unit, a ship, a lodge, a hospital.

To a lot of people, a chaplain is a man who "left the ministry," who couldn't make it, who got too old to be a pastor of a church, who couldn't preach good sermons—you name it.

To a Congregational minister named Anton Boisen, more than forty years ago, a chaplain looked like a man with possibilities:

—a specially trained minister in a hospital or prison

—a man who could understand people's problems

—a minister to people abandoned by their pastors and churches

—a man who could help doctors become more sensitive to the hurts their patients felt.

Boisen's first program for training chaplains has become a network of training centers all over the United States and Canada and is now spreading throughout the world.

To me, Chaplain Sam Perkins of Midbank University Hospital, a chaplain is a guy with a foot in two worlds: the world of faith and the world of modern medicine:

Not a doctor, but often asked to "explain" an operation.

Not a priest, but sometimes a baptizer of Catholic babies.

Not a social worker, but often a family counselor.

Not a professor, but on and off a teacher of young doctors.

Not a parish pastor, but usually a pastoral counselor.

In a society where medicine is more and more complex and impersonal, a man who sometimes can make the hospital seem more human.

Sometimes just a guy who listens over coffee to the bitching of a scared and exhausted young intern.

A man whose prayers are seldom uttered in the quiet of a church, but more often on the run, or down the hall, or as he hangs up the phone.

A man who can't ignore the special claims of his own church, who must wrestle with his own faith (and faithfulness), but . . .

A man who may have to minister to Baptists, Pentecostalists, Jews, Catholics, Presbyterians, and help them tussle with their own beliefs in the midst of crisis.

An impossible job?

Of course.

Maybe that's why he does it.

Perhaps all this sounds as if I'm trying to toot a horn, to say what a wonderful, marvelous, fantastic person a chaplain is. Perhaps trying to make it romantic.

That's why I haven't written this before now. I'm not a general hospital chaplain anymore; I'm a teacher. But I was chaplain of Midbank Hospital for several years, and I've let the experience simmer on the back burner, so that I could sort out what it meant.

As a chaplain I made dozens of mistakes, failed at all the tasks described above, succeeded at all of them, too. I learned from the physicians I worked with to take a really critical look at everything I did, to ask over and over again how it could have been done better. I know that there are competent chaplains and incompetent ones, men of faith and cynics, chaplains who are ministers and chaplains who are pseudo doctors, strong and weak men, men in the chaplaincy who chose an exciting and useful form of ministry and men who drifted into chaplaincy because they couldn't do anything else.

But that's true of parish ministers. And obstetricians. Surgeons. Lawyers. Architects.

The only special claim I want to make for chaplains is that their work is little known.

For more than six years I was chaplain of Midbank University Hospital. To everybody in a hospital—doctors, patients, admissions clerks, nurses—the place looks different. I know of a few books that describe a hospital from a physician's point of view, such as Michael Crichton's *Five Patients*, or Doctor X's *Intern*.

Of course, I think the chaplain's point of view is special because of his position on the boundary between patients and doctors, science and faith. This book is about how one chaplain worked, and how he saw one hospital.

II

A DAY

At Midbank University Hospital, Tuesday starts at about seven thirty Monday evening. That's when the surgical schedule for Tuesday is handed out. Charge nurses call it the "Daily Purple" because it's duplicated on a ditto machine, and they hate to see it coming. In the first place, it means work. In the second place, the work that the Daily Purple calls for can't be done unless a doctor orders it done. If Mr. Jones has chest surgery Tuesday at eight in the morning according to the Purple, Karen Benson knows that he must be NPO'd—but she can't NPO him unless a doctor gives the order. (NPO stands for *nil per orem,* which is Latin for "nothing by mouth." To "NPO a patient" means to remove all edibles and drinkables from the room and to put a sign "Nothing by mouth" on the door. The patient might vomit in surgery and choke to death.) In the third place, the schedule will probably be changed at the last minute, so Mr. Jones won't really go to surgery until eleven o'clock.

About an hour after the Daily Purple comes out, but sometimes *much* later, the anesthesiologist will show up to talk to the patients to whom she will administer anesthesia in the morning. At MUH (Midbank University Hospital), most of the anesthesiologists are women MD's. They're a pretty sensitive crew; the surgeons take great delight in teasing them. ("Hey, JoAnn, I hear you're gonna pass gas for me tomorrow.") The anesthesiologists prick up their ears when a patient begins to talk about dying in surgery. That's when Tuesday starts for the chaplain.

"Chaplain Perkins, this is JoAnn Sutherland. Do you know Mr. Frisbee on D-7?"

"No, can't say I do."

"Well, he's up for a TUR (trans-urethral resection, a prostate-gland operation) in the morning, and I've just been in to see him. Karen Benson said he seemed depressed, and I thought so too. He's sure he's going to die in surgery, and I smell a rat. Could you talk to him?"

"Glad to. D-7?"

"Right."

"Mr. Frisbee, I'm Chaplain Perkins. I hear you're going to have surgery tomorrow."

"Yes."

(The flat monosyllable, daring me to say anything.)

"Dr. Sutherland thought it might help if I talked with you about it."

"Nobody can help."

(Temptation. Reassure him, be cheerful. No, you know better.)

"She said you might feel that way, that you were pretty down."

"Guess I am. It's no use."

"You don't think things will go well tomorrow?"

"Depends on what you mean by 'go well.' "

"You have a hunch that you're going to die, don't you?"

Patients and chaplains sometimes seem to be the only people in hospitals who can use that word: die. Everybody else is part of a huge conspiracy. If they must say it, they say things like "slip away," "not make it," "go," or "expire."

"No hunch, I won't live through it. I know."

"Why is that?"

"It's my punishment. I've got it coming."

Slight sigh of relief. He has a reason. The scariest of all are the patients who "just know." Scary, because so often they *do* die. Tell an anesthesiologist or a surgeon that the patient thinks he's going to die "just because," and you get a nervous doctor. Sometimes they cancel the surgery.

"You believe that you're going to die tomorrow as a punishment. For what?"

"You ought to know; you're a chaplain."

"For your sins, then."

"Right. I'm a Christian. I know we have to pay for our sins."

"Is that what your church teaches, Mr. Frisbee?"

"They all do."

By now I am at a tough, important place. Just following his train of thought and reflecting his feelings seldom helps a depressed person. Reassuring him that everything will be all right is just plain foolish. The third choice—arguing with him —is something you seldom do. But in this case that third choice feels like the right one: not because his religious ideas are mistaken, but because stimulating a depressed man to express a little anger is the best way to start him out of his depression. Still, it's a risk.

"That hasn't been my experience, Mr. Frisbee."

"What do you mean?"

"Most churches I know teach that we *don't* have to pay for our sinfulness *that* way."

"You're kidding."

"Nope."

"But, I've committed adultery!"

(Here was another clue. The TUR, an operation on his genital-urinary system, might be connected with the fact that he was worrying about sexual behavior.)

"What did Jesus do with the woman taken in adultery?"

"I dunno. Forgave her?"

"Exactly."

"But my wife has never forgiven me. I can't forgive myself."

"You think your moral standards are higher than God's?"

"Of course not."

"That's what you just said."

"But I don't believe that!" (*By now indignant, a good sign.*)

"No, I don't think you really do. But that's what it means when you say that God will kill you tomorrow because you've committed adultery."

"Well, what about my wife?"

"Perhaps after your surgery you and your wife and I could talk about that."

"Do you think she would?"

"Do *you?*"

"Maybe she would. I'd like to try it."

"O.K. Tomorrow, while you're in surgery, I'll talk with your wife."

"That's great. Will you stop by and see me too?"

"You'll be pretty drowsy tomorrow, but I'll see you Wednesday."

"I'll count on that."

And that was the Monday night part of Tuesday.

What about Tuesday itself?

It began with an enraged internist. Edwin Holloman was a dirty-joke teller. He loved to stop in my office to see if he could shock me with a new one. He was also a lazy man. Whenever he had a patient who annoyed or troubled him, he'd simply book that patient into MUH. The house staff knew this and had it in for him. But there aren't too many ways a house officer can tell a senior staff member off.

As I walked into my office, there was Ed Holloman, his face the color of a ripe plum. To my greeting he simply growled an angry retort, and when I asked him what was wrong, he muttered that he was "going to get that smart-ass Bob Schumacher if it's the last thing I do!" And with that Ed stomped out.

I decided to start my rounds on D-7, hoping that I'd see Mrs. Frisbee, but also hoping that I'd see the medical resident on D-7, Dr. Bob Schumacher.

He was the first person I saw. Unshaven, obviously up all night, doggedly going through the charts of the forty-odd patients on his service.

"Hey, Bob."

"Hi, Sam."

"What in the world did you do to Ed Holloman?"

"Hot damn, he saw it!"

"Saw what?"

Grinning, Bob pulled out one of the rigid aluminum folders that contained a patient's chart.

"Read my admission note. It's Holloman's patient."

House officers learn to pack a great deal of information about a patient into the very first sentence of their writeups. A really good opening sentence will often tell the reader what the intern or resident is going to come up with as a diagnosis. Schumacher's opening sentence was a classic:

"This is the thirteenth MUH admission for this perfectly well fifty-nine-year-old white female infant, referred by Dr. E. Holloman."

I walk down the hall, threading my way among the breakfast carts. Benedict Martin, the priest from St. Mary Magdalen, walks toward me, head down. I almost say "Good morning, Ben," until I realize that he is carrying the Blessed Sacrament and will not speak.

It reminds me: the nurses often comment how unfriendly Father Martin is. He's not; he's a bouncy, friendly, cheerful man. But they see him only early in the morning as he brings Communion to Catholic patients. I've invited him to join the interprofessional seminar for house staff, nurses, and local clergy. Maybe that'll help.

I found Mrs. Frisbee weeping quietly in the D-7 waiting room.

Within a few minutes she was able to tell me how much she loved her husband, how angry she was with him, and how much she wanted to learn how to forgive him.

Our conversation was interrupted by the paging system: "Dr. Terman. Dr. Edgar Terman."

There was no Dr. Edgar Terman in the hospital. It was a code name to signal that the Emergency Room had an overload and that all available medical personnel were to report to the ER.

It also meant me.

When a large-scale emergency takes place, fifteen or twenty patients may be brought in at one time. For every patient brought in, there may be up to five relatives crowding the waiting room. The Emergency Room (ER) is laid out in such a way that the surgeons and nurses have to walk back and forth past the waiting room, and doing so, they collect anxious relatives the way a picnic collects ants. Their replies to questions become brusque and impersonal, because they are fully occupied with treating the maimed and identifying the dead.

I had discovered that a "Dr. Terman" call meant that the chaplain could be useful talking to relatives, keeping them away from the doctors, calming their fears, and sometimes staying with them when the news was bad.

This Tuesday, a school-bus driver, with his bus fully loaded, had collapsed at the wheel, letting his bus go out of control. The bus smashed into a culvert, injuring twenty-two children.

The waiting room was a babble of harried, distraught parents. Ann Robertson, the day head nurse, threw me a look of despair as I walked up to the desk.

"It doesn't matter where you start, Chaplain. They're all upset. But here's a list of injuries we've already treated. What'll I do?"

"I'll take the list. They probably need you back there."

O.K., Perkins, improvise.

"May I have your attention, please." (I had to repeat it four times before the room quieted down.) "Here is a list of the children who have been treated and will be released shortly. None of their injuries were serious."

There was a queer fascination in reading the list, watching some faces relax and others become more and more anxious as they did not hear the names they wanted to hear. I continued.

"This next group of children will all have to be admitted to the hospital. If one of your children's names is on this list, will you please step over to the clerk's desk? We'll need more information."

I finished the list. Almost home free. All broken bones. No life-threatening injuries for any child. Only one woman still stood there, her face now almost blank with dreadful knowledge. The bus driver's wife.

"What about my husband?"

"I don't know, ma'am, but I'll try to find out."

Threading my way down the hall to the last room, I found Ann Robertson pulling up a sheet over a face.

"The bus driver, Ann?"

"Yeh. Coronary. Menges just pronounced him, but he said the man was gone before the bus even hit the culvert. He never knew. Tell the wife?"

"I don't even know his name."

"Same as mine. Robertson."

(*Signal. Her father died of a coronary last month. See her after the crowd thins out.*)

"O.K."

Ordinarily, the chaplain isn't the person who tells family members that someone is dead. At MUH it is considered a doctor's job. It's important for house officers to learn to do this most disturbing of tasks. But this time it seemed right. The two Emergency Room interns were still sewing up cuts.

I went back to the waiting room.

"Mrs. Robertson?"

She froze. Not a muscle moved. I couldn't even see her mouth move, but words came out anyway.

"He's dead, isn't he?"

"I'm sorry, yes."

"Was it a heart attack?"

"The doctor thinks so."

Suddenly the frozen woman went from ice to steam. She screamed, collapsed on the floor, and lay there twitching. I heaved her onto a divan and grabbed Jim Menges, the intern who had pronounced her husband dead.

"That's Mrs. Robertson."

"I'll give her a sedative right away. Better get the black boy to carry her back to a bed."

Jim was from Alabama. Words like "black boy" crept into his speech only in emergencies. Bill Herman, the black aide, stood right behind him. Expressionless, Bill gently picked up Mrs. Robertson and put her on a cart as Menges went for medication.

Here was Ann Robertson again.

"Can you come sit with a frightened boy until the doctor gets to him?"

"Sure."

It was the last of the children from the bus accident, a big-eyed shivering boy with a nasty-looking laceration on his upper arm. He sat staring at the floor. During the ten minutes I stayed with him, he said not one word but looked up when I got a blanket to wrap around him. He followed me with his eyes as I left the room, kept watching me as I wrapped the blanket around him. When Jim Menges came in to dress the wound, the boy kept his eyes on me and wouldn't look at Jim. I almost couldn't walk out. I headed for the coffee shop.

Four interns were chuckling over Bob Schumacher's admission note on Ed Holloman's patient. Word gets around.

The page came on. "Chaplain Perkins, Chaplain Samuel Perkins." Reach for the phone. Dial zero.

"This is Chaplain Perkins."

"Dr. Gertner is looking for you. He's at the nurses' station on C-4."

Art Gertner was the chief of orthopedic surgery. He was a crackerjack surgeon but almost totally incapable of talking with patients. (So are lots of orthopedic surgeons. They have a reputation for being cold fish.) Art explained that a patient of his, a woman in her early thirties, had an osteogenic sarcoma—a form of bone cancer—in the tibia, the big bone of her lower leg. He would have to amputate the leg above the knee, but the woman wouldn't hear of it. Would I talk to her?

I went to the patient's room, thinking that Art had probably not explained the operation any too clearly. But when I arrived, I learned better. Throughout the visit the woman never stopped primping herself. She had decided not to have the operation, and that old Dr. Gertner (forty if he was a day) was just trying to mutilate her and get money for it. I listened for signs of the anxiety that must be there under all that vanity, but all I could hear was vanity. Either I was too angry or too tired to listen well. I prepared to take my leave.

"Chaplain"—seductively, like a little girl—"there is something you could do for me."

"Yes?" Was this a chance to help her?

"Would you please ask the nurse to go down to the gift shop and buy me some eye shadow?"

I had been betrayed by my Jesus complex, I told myself. You've got yourself convinced that you have to help every patient you see. Just like the damn doctors. Come on, Perkins, grow up. Give up. Let Gertner handle his own neurotics. Go to lunch.

Lunch with my friend Bill Hart, a psychiatric resident. He hadn't heard about the fifty-nine-year-old white female infant. I loved to hear Bill laugh.

Early afternoon. A marriage-counseling session with Jim and Sue Menges. The competent, confident, top-notch surgical intern now looks more like a confused, frightened child. Sue has worked throughout Jim's career in medical school. They celebrated Jim's graduation from med school by deciding to have a baby, and Sue quit her job as a nursing instructor three months ago. That much I know from just being around and chatting casually with Jim. What's gone wrong with their marriage, I don't know; this is their first session.

It turned out that the problem was a family problem. Jim's father, a small-town Alabama surgeon, wants Jim to take the rest of his residency in the South, closer to home, and then join him in practice. Sue has been putting pressure on Jim to take a residency here and to follow it up with an additional residency in thoracic surgery. Jim's just been sitting back and letting the two of them fight over him, and Sue is sick of it.

This case surely illustrates the dangers of referral. Fred Brenner, the Chief of Surgery, referred Jim to me. I'm pretty sure that Fred expects me to talk Jim into staying here for those residencies; he's had his eye on Jim for three months.

Odd, how a young doctor who's so decisive and courageous in his work is so passive and indecisive in his personal affairs.

Calls from patients.
Calls from doctors.
Calls from nurses.
The chaplain, like all hospital personnel, is at someone's beck and call. But there is one significant difference.
Initiative.
It's basically unethical for a doctor to start treatment without being asked. He's not supposed to take initiative in starting a relationship with a patient. But the chaplain *is*. For the chaplain to start a relationship isn't unethical at all. In addition to responding to requests from other professional personnel, the chaplain is at liberty to choose whom he will see and to use his own judgment in making choices of that kind.

Part of a chaplain's training consists of learning to make such judgments for himself.

Bill Breve, my opposite number at Wesley Hospital, tried to call on everybody every day. Some days that left him time to go back and see the people who looked as if they were in trouble. Other days, all he could do was wave hello to eight people at a time. I couldn't work that way.

I made heavy use of the nurses. I'd stop at the nurses' station on B-5 and ask Nan Johnson questions. Who's up for surgery tomorrow? Who's having trouble? Who's giving *you* trouble? Who's new?

I learned to ask more sophisticated questions. After reading Sidney Jourard's essay about nursing specialties, I learned to ask: What patients *haven't* you spoken to in the last eight hours? That way, I might discover the nurse's own hang-ups. I discovered from my own experience how right Jourard was. Some nurses just couldn't stop in to see a patient who wasn't going to recover. Other nurses like to spend loads of time with unconscious patients. Nan Johnson liked cantankerous patients and avoided the passive ones. Bea Williams avoided unwed mothers.

I could use my initiative to see just those patients it was hard for the nursing staff on a particular unit to work with. It created a kind of balance.

"Who's in trouble today, Miss Dill?"

"Oh, hi, Chaplain. No one, I guess. Well, maybe Miss Hulatz in 210. She just lies there. Medically, she's O.K. But she won't talk to anyone. Maybe there's a place to start."

"Well, I'll go see Miss Hulatz and check back with you when I'm through with her."

"Good."

Room 210 is a single room, quiet. Miss Hulatz lies on her back looking up.

"Good morning, Miss Hulatz. I'm Chaplain Perkins."

"I knew it."

"You knew I was Chaplain Perkins?"

"No. I knew I'd a need a chaplain. They lied to me, but I knew."

"When the chaplain comes in, you're sure it's really serious."

"Didn't Dr. Chasnoff send you?"

"No, he didn't. I came in on my own hook."

"Are you sure of that?"

"Yep, I'm sure."

"Well, they lied to me. They said my surgery went O.K., but I know I've got cancer."

"You believe that the doctors and nurses are deceiving you?"

"They're trying to. I had this operation, see, and they took a cancer out of my stomach. But now they're telling me it wasn't cancer."

"What is it that makes you sure it *is* cancer?"

"Well, my mother and my sister both died of cancer." (*And you lied to your mother, didn't you?*)

"Did they know they had cancer?"

"My mother didn't. We kept it from her. She thought she had pleurisy."

"So maybe they're keeping it from you—Is that what you think?"

"Sure."

"Must be pretty frightening, h'm?"

"Why won't they tell me the truth?"

"I'm not sure that's the problem. Maybe they are telling the truth."

"Well, if they are, what's the problem?"

"Looks to me like the problem is: Why can't you believe them?"

"That could be."

It took two more calls from me and a discussion with Dr. Isaac Chasnoff before the situation was resolved. I had to twist Dr. Chasnoff's arm a bit before he was willing to sit down with his patient. He was uncomfortable with patients, anyway. His habit was to examine Miss Hulatz' scar—which was healing nicely—and then back off, stand at the door, and exchange a few halting sentences with her. What he had a hard time seeing was that his manner was feeding Miss Hulatz' suspicions.

When he actually sat down by her bed to talk, she launched into an attack on him for lying to her. It took all his courage to stay sitting and fight it out with her. But when he was through, she seemed willing for the first time to believe that the big tumor he had removed from her abdomen really was benign.

She was still a little suspicious when she left the hospital.

But she wasn't killing herself psychologically.

The rest of the day was a mishmash, mostly calling on patients.

Even though I told Mr. Frisbee he'd be too drowsy after his

surgery for me to see him, I went up to the Recovery Room and checked, found him half awake, and dropped by D-7 to chat with his wife.

Then to D-4 to see a lady who had open-heart surgery a week ago. They called me to see her a couple of days ago when, like many open-heart patients, she became mentally ill. (It often happens, but the crazy thinking disappears after about forty-eight hours, as a rule.)

Stokeley, a medical intern, asked me to sit in with him while he tried to get a post permission from a very religious family. I never have figured out why fundamentalists are usually unwilling to let the doctors do an autopsy.

Ended the day at a CPC (Clinical Pathological Conference) where Phil Donnelly, an intern, had to listen to about seven senior staff members describe a case, and then tell them just from listening what the patient died of. It's like reading a detective story. All the clues are there, if you can just make them fit together. Being on the hot seat—that is, having Phil Donnelly's responsibility—is about as uncomfortable an hour as any intern ever spends, particularly with Bert Levine, the pathologist, making the final speech that tells the intern whether he was right or wrong. Phil was wrong today, and Levine cut him to shreds as usual.

They say it's the making of a doctor.

Tuesday's over. If JoAnn Sutherland runs into another problem tonight, she'll call one of the chaplaincy students in the clinical training program.

Tuesday's over.

It was an average day. I never did get back to Ann Robertson. Check on her tomorrow. No, I'll forget. She's still on duty down in the ER. Better stop by.

Tuesday isn't over.

Wednesday will start before Tuesday's over.

III
BIRTH

I HAD THE WRONG INTRODUCTION to obstetrics.

A premed friend of mine in college invited me to come with him to a meeting of the Pre-Medical Society. They had a movie on that night that was touted as GREAT! It was a film of a caesarian section, and the mother was carrying quadruplets.

The movie reminded me of one of those hand-quicker-than-the-eye magic tricks; it all took place so fast that I never really did see what happened. One midline incision from the navel to the pubic bone, and pop! There was a baby in the doctor's hands. So quick. So easy. And, on film, so impersonal.

It was no preparation for real obstetrics (OB), which is not quick, not necessarily easy, and not at all impersonal. A lot of hard work goes on in any hospital, but there's no place like a delivery room for giving you the sense of really hard physical work. No wonder they call it "labor."

Unlike surgery, obstetrics is loud. They yell, the obstetricians. "Come on, Emily, PUSH, dammit, PUSH!" The mothers aren't exactly quiet either.

Sometimes a hush does fall over the Delivery Room. The baby is born, is handed to someone, has his airway suctioned out, and is jolted into that first cry.

And the baby doesn't cry.

That's when things get pretty quiet.

It happens oftener than you'd think. But most of the time that first silence is eventually followed by a cry, and things get back to normally noisy.

The chaplain seldom goes into the Delivery Room. It's not really his work area; he has almost nothing to do there. But before he can work competently with obstetrical patients, the chaplain needs to have the delivery room experience under his belt. I always took my students in clinical training to see a delivery—and a surgical procedure, *and* an autopsy. They would never have any feeling at all for what it is like to be a doctor or a patient until they saw those procedures.

By the way, I never had a student faint while watching an autopsy or an operation. They usually didn't like watching and reported later that autopsies in particular were grim business —but they never passed out. But when we watched a delivery, I could always count on at least one student to sweat, to gag, or to crumple to the floor of the observation balcony.

Tim Logan, a young Catholic priest, explained it to me by quoting Latin: *"Inter faeces et urinam nascimur."* The other students, always impatient with Tim's pompous Latinisms, challenged him:

"O.K., Tim, say it in English."

"I'd rather not. You tell them, Sam."

"Nope, Tim, you said it, you translate it."

Flushing but determined, Tim translated: "We're born between the piss and the shit."

Is that the reason they faint? Because they realize for the first time what an earthy thing birth is? Death, by comparison, is so often quiet and sterile. Birth is noisy, full of fluids and excretions, and not a bit sterile. Is that what gets to them?

Seymour Grant was a young brain surgeon. His specialty, corrective surgery for very young babies—newborns, really— born with severe skull or brain problems.

Brian Terkelsen and Homer Trickett were medical students.

I saw them arguing angrily as I came through the lunch line in the hospital cafeteria, and I decided to join them.

"Hi, Chaplain."

"Hey, Chaplain, maybe you're the guy we ought to talk to about this."

"O.K., what's 'this'?"

Brian answered: "Well, Trick and I are on OB, and we saw something this morning. It's bothering us both."

"Yes?"

"Let me sum it up. We saw a baby born this morning with a bad skull defect. When the peds resident tried to start it breathing, it didn't go. Nothing. So, after that one slap, he looked at that skull and just gave up. Didn't try any more. Result was one dead baby."

"One dead glup, you mean. Why make a thing like that breathe when it'll probably die anyway, or be institutionalized all its life?"

"See what we mean, Chaplain? *I* say that they should have done everything they could to make that baby live; given it a chance. *Trick* says—well, you heard him."

"That's what you're arguing about?"

"Yeah."

"Well, look, here comes Dr. Grant. Let's get him in on this . . . Hey, Seymour, got a minute?"

Seymour Grant sat down and listened carefully to one more rehash of the argument between Terkelsen and Trickett. It didn't take him long to make up his mind.

"Of course you save the baby if you can. There's a lot we can do."

"Then you think it was wrong for the peds resident to give up?"

"Probably. I'll grant you, it may have been a baby with other defects, one that couldn't have lived. But you never know, that soon after birth."

"But, Dr. Grant, suppose you operate and save the baby's life, but it's essentially defective, would live as a vegetable for twelve years and then die. And somebody has to pay for the care for all those years. Why not just let the baby die?"

"You're playing God, Mr. Trickett."

"I don't know, sir." (*A bold young man!*) "Isn't it possible that by operating at all, *you*'re playing God?"

"Mr. Trickett, it's our calling to save lives wherever possible, under whatever circumstances. Better know that now, or you'll never be a doctor."

One year later.

Clover Myers is a woman, a physician, a resident in medicine, married to Seymour Grant, and pregnant. She is about to be pregnant no longer and is hard at work in the Labor Room. I saw her come in, smiling triumphantly and coping with her labor pains at the same time. She waved cheerily as they wheeled her past my office door toward the elevator.

About three hours later, as I was sitting in the corner of a waiting room, praying with a woman whose husband was in surgery, the paging system interrupted:

"Chaplain Perkins, Chaplain Samuel Perkins."

". . . Amen. Mrs. Elderby, would you excuse me, please?"

"Yes, sir. I'm feeling better now. You go on."

"Chaplain Perkins."

"Call 2513."

Dial.

"Delivery."

"This is Chaplain Perkins. Did you want me?"

"Oh, just a minute. Dr. Norris would like to speak to you."

"Sam!"

"Yes, Chet."

"Can you come up here on the double? You free?"

"What's up?"

"Well, pardon my French, but would you come up here and get that goddam Seymour Grant out of our hair? He's driving us crazy! Clover's in labor and doing fine, but a little slow. *He*'s pacing the hall, stopping every nurse. Can you come?"

"On my way."

Up on S-4, the obstetrical hall, I literally ran into Dr. Grant. He rounded a corner, half running, half walking, head down.

"Seymour!"

"Oh, hi. Clover's in labor. They say it'll be another hour. What's wrong?"

"Aw, c'mon, Seymour, even a chaplain knows that labor can last several hours. How about a cup of coffee?" (*Get him out of their hair is right. This zombi has forgotten everything he ever knew about medicine.*)

"Well, O.K. I'd like to talk to you anyhow."

"Something bothering you?"

"Yeah. Sam, it just occurred to me—What if the baby's deformed?"

"That worries you a lot, doesn't it? Maybe because you know more about deformations in newborns than anyone around here. You know too much, don't you?" (*I was leaping way ahead. Had I gone too far?*)

"Yeah. I know too much. Sam . . ."

"H'm?"

"If the baby *is* deformed . . ."

"H'm?"

"Maybe they should let it die."

Clover Myers Grant, M.D., was in labor eight hours. The baby was fine. So was Clover, and so was Seymour.

I see that I've left out the parts of those two stories that really have to do with the chaplain's work in the hospital. Not that having coffee with Seymour Grant, or putting the two young medical students in a position to talk with him, wasn't work. But the difficult work was helping the people involved to reflect on the religious and ethical issues. That's what a chaplain is there for, at least in part. Perhaps I've left that part out because it is so difficult, especially if you think there has to be a particular answer.

There isn't an answer: not one that will satisfy everyone. In the first place, the physician is trained to identify death or deformity or disease as *the* enemy to be overcome at all costs. Perhaps I've put that too strongly, but I don't think so. In the second place, there's a sense in which both Seymour Grant and Homer Trickett were right about playing God. Any time you practice medicine and take the responsibilities involved, you come into touch with that problem whether you try to save a newborn but damaged baby, or decide to let it go. Finally, you get to the point where you ask: Why? If you're a religious person—Christian, Jew, it doesn't matter—you may address your "why" to God. If you are not a believer, you still ask it, even though you're not talking to anyone in particular. One of my friends, a chaplain in an institution for retarded children, has only to look around him, and the "why" question comes up constantly. He rubs his students' noses in it. What is the meaning of the birth of defective, damaged, retarded children? How much control over such births and lives does the doctor dare exercise? Whether you are a physician or a chaplain, you wonder if you can explain it.

I don't think you can. You can't avoid wrestling with the mystery, but you can't expect it to be any less of a mystery no matter how much work you do on it. Anguished parents often ask if God is punishing them for their sins, a poignant reflection of that passage in the ninth chapter of John's Gospel when the disciples asked Jesus whether a man born blind had himself sinned or if the fault was that of his parents. Doctors often seem to try to live by Jesus' answer, even if they are not religious men themselves: "It is not that this man or his parents sinned. . . . While daylight lasts we must carry on the work." (John 9:3-4, NEB.) You do what you know how to do.

You try to salvage deformed babies because those are the talents God has given you; but you still have your doubts and fears, even about your own child. Or you look at a baby who won't (can't? shouldn't?) breathe in the Delivery Room, and you put him down gently, still not breathing, never to breathe.

And you wonder if you've done the right thing, but you go right on to the next delivery and work (sweat!) to make *that* baby breathe.

Word about unusual births gets around the hospital quickly. There was a Thursday morning when five times in the space of an hour, somebody told me of the professor's wife who had had triplets. The nurses were excited, the doctor was secretly pleased, and the father was proudly handing out three cigars at a time—all because a zygote had split in an unusual way. (A zygote is the first cell of the new baby formed at conception. Some multiple births stem from the splitting of the zygote into separate cells.) Sandy Bird, one of the nurses on the night shift in OB, left a note for me saying that the mother seemed to be unhappy, maybe depressed.

I seldom called on the mothers who had had normal uncomplicated deliveries. It was a luxury I couldn't afford. Occasionally I'd give myself the pleasure of rejoicing with the rejoicing parents, but the problems and the crises seemed to be the places where a chaplain was more needed. (Today, I'm not so sure about that.)

But here was an instance in which it might be appropriate to stop by. I knew Stan and Muriel Baker slightly. Stan taught political science at Midbank University. If Muriel was depressed, it might be important to see if the depression was just a response to suddenly having three babies, or whether some more serious problem was in the wind, in which case a psychiatric consultation could be appropriate. So I stopped by to see Muriel.

When she recognized me, she burst into tears.

"Sam, how am I going to cope?"

"Three children are a lot, aren't they, Muriel?"

"Oh, God, yes. Why didn't Carl know ahead of time?" (Carl Teague, her obstetrician, had apparently not predicted the multiple birth.)

"I couldn't say. I don't know how easy or hard it is for doctors to predict those things ahead of time. I know that sometimes they can. Sounds like you're kind of angry at Carl."

"Oh, I know, I shouldn't be. But my Lord, Sam, there were two of us and we'd planned for three of us and now there're five of us. I can't take care of three babies all at once. Our parents are both dead, and I can't afford to hire help on an assistant professor's salary. It's just too much. And that Stan . . ."

"Angry with him too?"

"You betcha. He's so pleased about it, he hasn't come down to earth yet. He doesn't even realize what it's going to mean for us. The work, the money problems, three kids in diapers: I'll have to deal with all of that all by myself."

"You really feel that Stan doesn't realize what it's going to mean, and you'll have the entire burden."

"Oh, yes. It's going to be just terrible."

(*Again the temptation. Tell her it won't be terrible. Try to get her to see the bright side. Then the wiser voice: That's what everybody's been saying to her, and it just makes her more depressed.*)

"You're afraid you can't hack it, aren't you?"

The day charge nurse, Frances Adams—known to all as Fussy Fanny—bustles in.

"Oh, Chaplain, Mrs. Baker isn't allowed to have visitors. You'll have to leave."

"If he goes, I go."

"Whaaaat?"

"You people make me sick! I don't need your protection! I'll see who I want to see!"

"You see, Chaplain, Mrs. Baker isn't quite herself. Now if you'll just—"

"No, Sam, don't go. I need to talk with you."

"Muriel, I'll be back in a little while. Hang on."

Sweet Fanny Adams and I step out into the hall.

"Miss Adams, I don't want to discuss this with you in front of Mrs. Baker. If you'd like, we can call Dr. Teague and check this out. I did stop at the desk and check with Mrs. Wilson before I called on Mrs. Baker, as a courtesy to you all."

"Now, Chaplain"—explaining to a little child—"you should know better. Dr. Teague said No Visitors."

"If I'm included in that, so are the aides, the housemaids, and the nurses, Miss Adams. You need to understand that I'm a member of the hospital's professional staff: NOT A VISITOR!"

(How did I get into this childish battle? I'm fighting on her terms.)

"I'm going to call Dr. Teague."

"Fine. Let me know how it comes out. I'll be with Mrs. Baker."

Back into the room.

"Oh, Sam, I'm so sorry."

"Don't take on that burden too, Muriel. I just wanted to say that I'll stop by again this afternoon when Stan is here. I think we need to talk together."

"Oh, would you? Sam, before you go . . ."

"Would you like a prayer?"

"Yes, please."

I prayed for strength and maturity—Muriel's and mine.

On the way out, I stopped at the nurses' station. Miss Adams looked up.

"Did you talk with Dr. Teague?"

"Yes."

"What did he say?"

"He said that you could call on any of his patients any time. But, Chaplain, I'm going to have to take this up with Dr. Norris."

"Of course."

One small victory, one new enemy. Lord, help me to deal with crap like that more wisely.

At MUH, mothers who had lost their babies roomed together. The idea, of course, was that no woman who had lost a baby should be subjected to the sight of watching another mother caring for her own squalling bundle of life. It was probably a wise policy.

The trouble was that many of the OB nurses avoided the rooms where the bereaved mothers were. Sidney Jourard, a psychologist in Florida, once wrote a beautiful paper about nursing specialties. He pointed out that some nurses specialize in dealing only with people who can be cured or with properly married mothers—in other words, with people they could be comfortable with. I think Jourard was right. One young nurse confessed as much one day: "I don't know what to say to those poor women who've lost their babies, Chaplain."

"It *is* tough, isn't it? But, you know, Sue, I wonder if it might not be pretty tough for those mothers to feel that they're not able to talk to people either. Maybe they feel that they're getting just the minimum of attention."

"I guess so, Chaplain. And maybe that makes them feel even more like failures."

"Maybe it does at that."

And Sue went into the mothers-without-children room, perhaps to try once more.

IV
CHILDREN

CHILDREN HAVE FEELINGS.

Adults have feelings.

Adults often think that they're paying attention to children's feelings when they're really only paying attention to their own feelings.

That's what makes pediatrics a difficult service.

On a really good pediatrics service there is a constant tension between paying attention to the needs and feelings of the children, on the one hand, and doing the very adult, careful, technical procedures that children may or may not understand, on the other. The younger the child, the more this tension becomes apparent.

Why? Because the smaller a child is, the harder it seems to be for adults to understand what his needs and feelings are; but the smaller a child is, the more important it becomes to be very careful and precise with the technical things you do. (A slight change in medication makes a bigger difference in a small body.)

In the mid-1950's a group of medical students at Washington University School of Medicine put on a show in which they teased the pediatrics professor with the lines:

> Twenty cc's of sugar per kilogram,
> Weigh the feces to the nearest milligram.

That kind of careful measurement really is important in pediatrics.

In dealing with the needs of children, hospitals make mistakes in two ways.

One way is to isolate the child, particularly from his parents. That doesn't happen much in American hospitals, and hasn't for a long time. But until very recently, the British did it that way, until a series of studies made it clear how cruel and unthinking and *detrimental to recovery* it is to prohibit contact between sick children and their parents. Even then, it took a long time for British hospitals to change. (Some of that struggle is reflected in a book called *Children in Hospital.*)

The other mistake is to adopt the "poor little thing" approach that treats the child as an object of pity to be coddled and catered to at every turn. Maybe that approach, by generating our feelings of pity for sick children, raises money. It surely turns on feelings—including mine—to see a sick child, or a child on crutches. But those are *our* feelings, and they aren't the children's feelings.

Parents are often the worst offenders. (Maybe that explains why British hospitals took the attitude they did.) Parents often feel guilty about a sick or crippled child, as if it had been the mother's carelessness or lack of love that got the child into this mess. Mama is busy trying to make up for the past, but little Pete, four years old, is just interested in trying to make things go better now and in the future.

MOTHER: Oh, poor little Petey, Mother will help you use your crutches. Here, let me hold you up.

PETEY: Mother, please! I'd rather do it myself!

If Petey can't say that to his mother—and he often can't —it may be the nurse or the aide who has to uphold Petey's side of things. Mother, of course, will think that the nurse is cold and hard. But it's the nurse who is paying attention to Petey's feelings—and contributing to his recovery.

Nothing outside of good technical medical care will speed recovery faster than a thoughtful, supportive mother who really wants the child to become strong, well, and independent. And nothing slows recovery more than a guilty mother who tries to make the child dependent on her for everything.

End of sermon.

I'd stuck my head in to see eight-year-old Bill Pardue, who was going down for catheterization later that morning. (Before heart surgery, the surgeon has to try to find out what the heart and blood vessel structures are like inside the patient's chest. So a team inserts a thin tube—a catheter—into a vein and runs it on into the heart. Carefully. It's painful sometimes, and dangerous. But it's necessary.) Billy was doing fine, but as I left the room Milly Trader, one of the nurses, got up from her charts and stood there trembling.

"Chaplain Perkins . . ."

"Morning, Miss Trader."

"There's a child I'd like you to see, a house-staff patient."

Tears ran down her cheeks. Not like tough, self-contained Miss Trader.

"What's the problem?"

"Burns. But what's getting me is how he got those burns."

"What do you mean?"

"Well, they just brought him in from the ER. I think his father did it to him deliberately. Pete Winthrop got a little history, and the mother said that the kid 'fell' into a tub of scalding water."

"You don't believe it?"

"Oh, God, Chaplain, no. Nobody's talked to the child. He's obviously scared to death."

"What's his name?"

"Jimmy Dunn. Oh, Chaplain, thank you."

(*See the cool, businesslike chaplain asking questions. See how competent and professional the chaplain is. See the chaplain who isn't sure if or how he can help. The chaplain is praying. He is saying, "O Lord, what am I doing here?"*)

"Hello, Jimmy."

He is trembling. Is it the burns, or is it something else?

"Who are you?"

"I'm the chaplain. I came to see how you were doing."

"What's a chaplain?"

"A minister."

"Like in our church?"

"Kind of like that. What happened to *you?*"

"I was a bad boy." (*Try to remember, Perkins, what your old supervisor said about talking to children. What does he mean, "bad boy"?*)

"I don't think I understand." (*At least you can be honest.*)

"Daddy says I'm punished for my sins."

"You mean the burns?"

"Yes, sir."

"Burns are a punishment?"

"I was playing in the bathroom, and I shouldn't've. I fell into the water, and it was hot." (*It sounds rehearsed, unbelievable.*)

I look around, aware of a presence. Milly Trader is standing there. I get the feeling she wants to be a witness to what's said.

"How old are you, Jimmy?"

"Six."

"In the first grade?"

"Yes, sir."

"Well, how does a big six-year-old boy fall into a bathtub?" (*Careful. Don't ask a child too many questions, or ones he can't answer.*)

"I don't know." (*But you know he does know. What's stopping him?*)

"Are you scared, Jimmy?"

"Yes." A whisper.

"Miss Trader and I would like to help you be less scared. Can you tell us about it?"

"Will you tell my mommy and daddy?" (*A crucial point. If you say yes, he may not say anything. If you say no, it might be a promise you couldn't keep. You could even get into legal trouble.*)

"No." (*You've crossed over. No going back now.*)

"Daddy put me in the tub. He said I was bad and he was going to wash me clean of my sins." (*Oh, God! Half swearing, half praying. A thickness in my throat. I'm going to vomit. I'm going to have loose bowels. I'm going to wet my pants. See the professional chaplain.*)

"Jimmy, I'll bet it hurts a lot."

"Yes, sir."

"Well, Miss Trader and the doctors are going to make you feel better."

"Sir?"

"H'm?"

"Are my sins washed away now? Does God love me again?" (*Oh, Jimmy.*)

"They sure are. God does love you, Jimmy."

"That's good."

And where do you get off, Sam Perkins, telling him that God loves him? You know damn well he means his father. You can't tell him his father is sick in the head. You're telling a truth and a lie at the same time.

"Chaplain Perkins . . ."

"Yes, Miss Trader?"

"If I write this up verbatim, will you sign it?"

"Yes, I'll sign it."

And will Daddy get treatment, or will he just go to jail?

Religious issues come up in dozens of unexpected ways on pediatrics.

"Chaplain, there's some kind of nutty evangelist up here! He's got a little pulpit set up in the hall and is preaching to the kids that they must be saved before they die." (Chaplain's task: get him out of there.)

"Chaplain, some of the nurses have been wondering if we could have a Sunday school for the kids." (Help the nurses to find another way to channel those good intentions, because the hospital has to stay neutral.)

"Chaplain, we've just had to tell a couple that their child has leukemia, and they're pretty broken up about it. Can you come up?" (. . . and help them handle their feelings?)

"Chaplain, there're some people up here who won't let us give their child a blood transfusion. They say it's against their religion." (Yes. Jehovah's Witnesses, who believe that to accept a blood transfusion is literally to lose your chance for heaven. Task: to help the staff understand the facts, to help them decide whether they want to make a court case out of it.)

"Chaplain, there's a lady up here who is going up and down the halls asking other parents if their children are going to die." (And so, Chaplain, will you get her off people's backs? *She's* not a patient, so we can't ask for a psychiatric consultation.)

"Chaplain, what do we do about a Catholic child who is dying?" (Answer: I'll call Father Martin of St. Mary Magdalen parish. He'll be able to decide what's appropriate.)

"Chaplain, there's a child up here who won't eat. He says the food's not kosher." (Answer: Technically, an orthodox Jew in the hospital is excused from keeping kosher. But the kitchen has kosher diets, and the boy's parents could ask the doctor if it'd be all right to put the boy on a kosher diet.) Interestingly, the boy who as a Jew won't eat nonkosher food and the Jehovah's Witnesses who won't permit blood transfusions are basing their beliefs on the same passage in the Old Testament. Slightly different traditions, though.

One day—one night, really—Sue Puckett, the night charge nurse, asked me to come in and talk with a pair of disturbed parents. From that eerie, brightly lighted hall into the dark (one sixty-watt bulb) of a waiting room, to find Mr. and Mrs. Murphy sitting dully in a corner, not looking at each other.

"Are you the Murphys?"

"Yes, sir."

"I'm Chaplain Perkins."

"What denomination are you, Chaplain?"

"Reformed Church."

"Well, we're Babdists. Up here from Tennessee."

"Did you have a religious question?"

"Well, yessir, we did. Y'see, our boy Danny has leukemia, and the doctors tell us they ain't no chance for him to live."

"That must be a hard blow to take."

"Well, it *is*. What makes it so bad, we done it."

"You mean you gave the child leukemia?"

"In a way. See, Danny's our only, and, well, sir, we ain't really married."

"I don't quite understand." (*Actually, I think I do.*)

"We've been livin' together, what's the word the doctor used?"

"Common law?"

"Yessir, common law, and so Danny was born in sin. We figure that the Lord's punishin' us for our sins. Don't seem quite right, though."

"How's that?"

"Killin' the tyke for what *we* done."

"Mr. Murphy, how long have the two of you been living together?"

"Sixteen years."

"Do you take care of Mrs. Murphy and Danny?"

"What do you mean, mister? He sure does. Been as good a man to me and Danny as any woman'd ever want."

"So the two of you have been trying to make a good home for yourselves and Danny?"

"Yessir. Twelve years before he come along, and four years since."

"He's a *good* man, Chaplain."

"I'm sure he is, Mrs. Murphy. In fact, I just wonder . . ."

"What's that?"

"Well, it seems to me that you've been trying to live a good life, provide a home, rear Danny right, and things like that."

"Well, sir, we've tried."

"But what you're worried about is that by not getting a license and going before a preacher you've done something terribly wrong."

"Guess so. That's why Danny's dyin'."

"Do you really think a loving God would punish you that way? One mistake sixteen years ago and trying to live right, do right, ever since?"

"Well, Chaplain, would you marry us?" (*Careful, Perkins!*)

"I think the two of you *are* married in every sense but legally."

(*They're probably even married legally.*)

"But would you marry us? We got a license yesterday . . ."

"Yes, Mrs. Murphy, I would if that's what you wanted. But there's more to it than that."

"What's that?"

"I wonder if you're perhaps thinking that if I married you, it would make Danny get better?"

"Well . . ."

"You did have that hope, didn't you?"

"Guess so."

"Mrs. Murphy, Danny has a very serious disease. He really didn't get it because you have a common-law marriage, and changing it to a legal marriage with papers and preachers and all won't get rid of the disease. Do you know what I'd say to you in a wedding ceremony?"

"Kind of."

"Well, I'd ask you, Mr. Murphy, if you'd be a loving and faithful man to Mrs. Murphy here, and you'd say yes, wouldn't you?"

"Course."

"But you've *been* a loving and faithful man to her for sixteen years."

"And I've been loving and faithful to him, mister."

"Exactly. The Lord sees your mistake, but he also sees the

way you've been treating each other and Danny, and that's important."

"Well, then, why is Danny going to die?" (*There it is: the question they've really been wrestling with.*)

"I don't know. I don't know why he has that disease. But my church doesn't teach that it's because you lived together without being married, and neither does yours."

"It don't? Are you sure?"

"Yes, ma'am, I'm sure. If you've got any doubts, I'd be glad to get Brother Akers from the Lawndale Baptist Church over here to talk to you about it."

"Naw, that ain't necessary. If you're sure . . ."

"I *am* sure. But I can't answer that other question about why Danny has leukemia. That's an awful mystery."

"Well, what can we do?"

"What you can do is go right on loving and caring for Danny, just as you've always done. If he's going to be sick—and it looks like he is—then he'll need your love and care more than ever."

"Guess that's right, LouAnn."

"Guess it is, Billy Dee."

How did that go, Perkins? Did you help them? Did you do it right? Well, you were a little too intellectual, too logical. You maybe didn't deal with their feelings enough. You were a little too sure about what Willie Akers would say. But on the other hand you got them started thinking about what they could do for their sick son. And maybe they've begun to realize that they didn't make the boy get leukemia. All in all, though, too much rational, logical, theological stuff, and not enough dealing with their fear.

And you never asked them how Danny might have felt. Our feelings, our thoughts, not the child's thoughts and feelings. It's hard to keep remembering that. Tomorrow, see Danny Murphy and try again.

V

MEDICINE

EDDIE GROSSMAN was a bubbly pip-squeak of a medical intern whose cheerful, apparently superficial approach to everything hid a brilliant mind. The assistant residents referred to him as the Boy Diagnostician, in grudging appreciation of his powers at figuring out what was wrong with people. I enjoyed eating lunch at a table where Eddie sat. Good humor seemed to flow all around the table.

"Hey, Chaplain Sam, siddown! Hey, didja hear what happened in the ER this morning?"

"No, what?"

"Well, this big ol' black mama came in, see, and she wan't feeling any too good. They assigned Clem Skinner to pick her up, and he went out to the waiting room, and he said, 'I'm Doctor Skinner,' and ol' mama said: 'Just a minute! Is you a thinkin' doctor or is you a cuttin' doctor? "

We all laughed. I decided not to tell Eddie that "what happened in the ER this morning" was actually a classic story told as true in dozens of teaching hospitals around the country.

There's a long-standing and sometimes even useful rivalry between medical and surgical services. The surgeons call the medical men "pill-pushers" and the medics call the surgeons "barbers." Medical staff love to quote Sir William Osler: "If the patient is improving, change nothing; if the patient is getting worse, change everything; and never call the surgeon."

(That's how I heard the quotation; I've never looked it up.) My own feelings gradually took the form of saying to myself that the surgeons changed what couldn't be managed, and the medics managed what couldn't be changed.

What impressed me most of all about the medics—by the way, they are the men who would be called internists when their residencies were completed—was how much work they had to do in teaching their patients to manage themselves, particularly in chronic illnesses such as heart disease, diabetes, or emphysema.

At seven thirty every morning a messenger from the Admissions office slid an A & D sheet (a dittographed record of all Admissions and Discharges from one midnight to the next, distributed to just about everyone in the hospital) under the door of my office. I'd routinely pick it up off the floor as I walked in, and it was the first thing I looked at to start my day. Who expired yesterday? Who's gone home? Who's here?

It was a bright August Monday, promising that baking Midwestern heat, when, as I scanned Sunday's A & D sheet my eye was caught by a new medical admission: "Shelton, F. K." Could it be Kilby Shelton? Could it be the Reverend F. Kilby Shelton IV, D.D. "Luh-huv" of God Shelton?

Kilby Shelton was the pastor of the largest church in town: 3,500 communicant members, a staff of fifteen permanent employees. Perhaps I should say semipermanent. No assistant pastor stayed there any longer than he could help. Kilby had his own television program, where he preached insistently, cheerfully, aggressively about the luh-huv of God. I had to admit to myself that he wasn't my favorite clergyman, particularly since he had the habit of interfering with patient treatment, suggesting to the doctors that they didn't know what they were doing. He consistently advised bereaved families that they should refuse permission for postmortem examinations, managing to suggest subtly that such an examination was against the religious beliefs of The Methodist Church. (It isn't.)

The A & D sheet listed "Shelton, F.K." as a patient in a private room on F-6. I decided I'd call on him later in the morning.

"Why, hello there, Sam!"

"Hello, Kilby. I saw your name on the list of admissions this morning and thought I'd drop by."

" 'Preciate it."

"What brought you in?"

His voice—oh, cliché—sank to a conspiratorial whisper.

"Well, I've just come in to get regulated."

"Diabetes?"

"You guessed it. Yep, Dr. Cargo wants to change my medication a little bit. A little more insulin."

"Well, I didn't know you were a diabetic."

"Well, you know, it's not the kind of thing you tell people."
(*Isn't it? Most diabetics learn not to make a secret of their condition, particularly since they may need emergency treatment at almost any time.*)

"You'd really rather not have people know?"

"You know how people are, Sam. I'll trust you not to say anything."

"O.K. I see your doctor is Prez Cargo. O.K. if I mention to him that I've seen you?"

"Why, of course, my boy. But there's nothing to worry about, you know. Just a little matter of regulation of the insulin. Glad you dropped by." (I had been dismissed, and I knew it.)

In the hall later, here comes rumpled Prez Cargo in his yesterday's clothes.

"Hi, Prez."

" 'Lo, Sam."

"Prez, I saw Kilby Shelton earlier today."

"Good. Think you can help him?"

"Why, what's to help?"

"Didn't read the chart, did you?"

"I confess, officer."

"Read the charts, boy!" (Why was it that when Prez Cargo said "boy" I felt good but from Kilby Shelton it was such an insult?)

"Seriously, Sam, I think you could help the Reverend Shelton. He's got a terrible problem."

"He said he came in for adjustment of his insulin."

"He came in out cold in a diabetic coma. I'm surprised he was awake when you saw him. They brought him in through Emergency."

"Prez, are you saying it's a long-range problem? Poor control of his diabetes?"

"Man's a pig. He'll clean the trough and squeal for more."

"I noticed he seemed to need to keep his condition quiet."

"Well, that's part of the problem too. Doesn't want anybody to know. Part of why he overeats, maybe. He'll never have insulin shock that way. And insulin shock's so much more noticeable than going down gradually into a coma the way he does."

"Has he been in a coma before?"

"Several times. His heart's affected, and his eyes. I'd say we've got a frightened man, but is he frightened enough to do something about it this time? Imagine Shelton as an amputee, Sam."

"I get the picture. I'll try to talk with him."*

The next day, I stopped in to see Kilby Shelton again.
"Hello, Kilby."

---

* Perhaps this conversation needs a little explaining. In diabetes, the chemical compound (insulin) that neutralizes unused sugar in the blood either isn't present or doesn't work. Sugar levels in the blood rise too high (hyperglycemia), producing eventual coma and death. Hyperglycemia can affect the circulation, producing gangrene, heart trouble, eye trouble, and other problems. Insulin can be given by injection. Together with a properly controlled diet, this will produce a more normal blood sugar level. If you burn up too much sugar and fail to eat, a low blood sugar level (hypoglycemia) results, producing what is often called insulin shock. Quick administration of sugar by oneself or others can reverse the shock effect. Insulin shock comes on quickly, as a rule.

"Hi, there."

"You're looking good." (*Too good. You're over the coma, and you're not going to be concerned enough.*)

"Feelin' fine. Imagine Doc Cargo will let me go home tomorrow."

"Yes. Kilby . . . you didn't just need adjustment, did you?" (*Make it a direct attack, Perkins.*)

"What do you mean?" suspiciously.

"I mean you came in in a coma through the Emergency Room."

"How did you know?"

"It's on the admission sheet." (*It was. I hadn't noticed at first.*)

"Oh. Well, that's all over now."

"Is it really? How well are you managing your diabetes?"

"Not as well as I might, I suppose."

"So you might go into a coma again."

"Aw, no. I've sworn off eating."

"That isn't going to be enough, is it?" (*This man will have to be approached directly. How can I get through if Prez hasn't?*)

"You mean I don't keep my promises?"

"How many times have you sworn off eating before?"

"This time I mean it."

"Kilby, you are talking like an alcoholic. That's what *they* say."

"Get out of here! Get out!"

"Not until I've finished. This once you're not like the centurion who says 'Go!' and people go. You're a sick man and you've got a disease that can be controlled and you're not controlling it. Do you know what you are?" (*Lord, Perkins, you're scolding the most respected pastor in town.*)

"What?"

"You're a poor steward."

"I don't understand." (*Have I got his attention with that word?*)

"I've heard you talk about stewardship, using and caring
for the things God's placed in your care. Well, what kind of
steward of your body are you?"

"You're right. You're right."

And the Reverend F. Kilby Shelton, D.D., started to cry.

I went away feeling that it was a poor interview. I'd scolded,
I'd used a religious idea that got his attention, but when he
cried I softened up, forgetting that he really was like an alcoholic, and that the crying was a defense against the work he
needed to do, just as his "swearing off" had been.

Later, I talked again with Prez Cargo. He was intrigued by
the parallel to alcoholism and decided that Marie Shelton,
Kilby's wife, would have to be enlisted. Prez, a dry alcoholic
himself, got Marie to promise that if Kilby ate himself into a
coma again, she'd leave him—*and* he got her to promise to tell
Kilby that.

Kilby denounced doctors and MUH from his pulpit.

Then he ate himself into a coma.

When he had pulled through, Marie left him. She wrote him
a note saying she'd come back when he'd lost forty pounds.
(Prez's idea.)

He lost the weight.

Marie came back.

Throughout that period, Prez Cargo and I kept telling each
other that we were doing the right thing.

I still think the stewardship idea was right. And I still think
I misused it.

Bald, dapper little Perce Crosby stopped in my office on his
way out of the hospital. Perce was an internist in town, and a
good one. He'd had his residency at MUH and now was one of
the attending physicians. He was always friendly but seldom
stopped in unless there was a specific problem—so I wondered
just what he wanted as he fenced around being friendly. Finally it came.

"Sam, I've got a patient I'd like you to see."

"O.K. (I chuckled to myself, because I knew that Perce would talk like a medical chart.)

"This is the second MUH admission for this twenty-year-old girl. Her chief complaint was itching, and I noticed enlarged lymph nodes in her neck. That is a classic indication of lymphadenoma or Hodgkin's disease, so I had her admitted for a lymph node biopsy and other diagnostic studies. It's Hodgkin's, all right. I'm sure. I told her this morning, and she was pretty frightened. You know, there are all kinds of possibilities, and some of these Hodgkin's patients survive a very long time. But I told her I thought it was unwise for her to have any children, and that disturbed her severely."

"Perce, what would you like me to do?"

"Well, it occurred to me that you might provide some support for her in this difficult period. She is very religious, belongs to one of the conservative sects, I believe."

"How much have you predicted, Perce?"

"I gave her a pretty thorough rundown on what she might expect: long survival, short survival, spiking fevers. But she didn't hear it much. I think she thinks she's going to die rapidly, and that's not necessarily the case at all. You know?"

"I think I understand. With a little support she might be able to resume a relatively normal life?"

"Oh, I think so. I must go. Will you see her?"

"Gladly." (*Hah! After a while I begin to talk just like him.*)

"Miss Perkins, I'm Chaplain Perkins."

"Oh, we have the same name, don't we?"

"Looks like it."

"Do you call on all the patients in the hospital? You must be very busy." (*Is she putting me off?*)

"No, I don't see all the patients. Many of them have their own pastors coming, and many of them don't feel any need to see a chaplain. I came to see you because Dr. Crosby mentioned you to me."

"Why did he do that?"

"Well, I think he thought that he'd given you some pretty bad news, and that you might like to talk about it."

"I guess I would, at that. How much time do you have?"

"Well, about twenty minutes right now, but I can come as often as we think it might be useful to talk."

"Well, it's this way. With only a year or so to live, I want to get out of here and go do some living. I've been a goody-goody all my life, and I'd like to live before I die."

(*Surprise, surprise!*)

"Sounds like you feel you haven't got much time." (*Now I see the meaning of her question about how much time I have.*)

"I don't, do I?"

"And so you want to kick over the traces, sow some wild oats?"

"Right!"

Now I had a whole collection of feelings and hunches. The most likely one was that this girl with such a religious and conservative background was furious at God for her disease and was going to express the anger with a little high living. I also hunched that if she did so, she'd become very guilty and depressed. I couldn't test all that out in a twenty-minute talk, so . . .

"Miss Perkins, I'm finding myself wondering if you feel pretty angry about this whole thing."

"Angry? No. Well, a little maybe."

"Maybe you'd like to talk about that."

"Well, I think I would."

"What angers you the most?"

"The fact that I can't have children. Dr. Crosby says I might not live to see them grow up. And I'm engaged to get married in the fall."

"You'd planned on children, and losing that really hurts."

"It does. How do I tell Al?"

"Telling your fiancé 'no children' is going to be hard."

"Could you be here when I tell him?"

"I don't see why not. Maybe we could all talk about your future."

"I think we ought to call off the wedding."

"Right now you think getting married would be unfair to Al?"

"Well, don't you think so, with me dying in a year or so?"

"You know, Miss Perkins, that's not what the doctor says." (*Now drop the Carl Rogers stuff.*)

"What do you mean?"

"Dr. Crosby told me that many patients with Hodgkin's disease live a very long time. Didn't he tell you that?"

"Maybe he did. I don't know."

"Do you suppose there's some reason why you might not have heard him?"

"Do you mean because I'm so mad and upset?"

"That's one possibility."

"Well, I feel so attacked!"

"You are attacked. You are attacked by a disease that may in time be fatal. What do you want to do about it?" (*You shift gears. You get tough, demanding. If you don't, she may die sooner than she needs to.*)

"You can't ask me to do anything about it!"

"I can and I do. This disease may kill you in five years or in thirty years. Whether it does the one or the other depends on you." (*In saying this, I still wonder how tough to be.*)

"You'd better go away and let me think about that."

"O.K. But I'll be back."

The next day.

"You're right, Chaplain Perkins. Only, y'know, I'd put it a different way."

"I'd like to know how you would put it."

"I'm going to be discharged tomorrow. I could get hit by a car on my way to the parking lot if I'm not careful. How I die is partly up to me."

"That's a good way to put it."

"And I'm going to get married *and* I'm going to have children."

Today Mary Perkins Crumley has
—Hodgkin's disease
—a child
—and a chance to live twenty more years.

A hot summer afternoon. A-3, one of the Women's Medicine wards, has never been air-conditioned. You stick to the chairs. You drip sweat onto beds.

I am sitting in a room where Mrs. Estelle Marcus, age seventy-three, is about to die. Her family has asked for me to be with them. They are moaning aloud, weeping, cracking their knuckles. Mrs. Marcus is breathing a la Cheyne-Stokes.* People reach out and squeeze my arm. I touch them. I'm conscious of the wetness.

The raspy breathing stops. Mrs. Marcus has died. We all know it, and moving as if we were one person, we stand up.

I ask: "Would you like me to have a word of prayer with you?"

The answer comes.

"Why, no, Mr. Perkins. Whatever in the world gave you that idea? Mother's gone; you can leave now."

*Ite Missa est.***

---

* Cheyne-Stokes breathing. Irregular breathing, unrhythmic breathing; first slow and shallow, then more rapid and deep, then slow again, then no breathing at all for several seconds. Then the cycle starts again. Cheyne-Stokes breathing often precedes death.
** "Go, it is the dismissal." The last words of the Roman Catholic Mass, from which, as a matter of fact, the Mass gets its name.

VI
SURGERY

BEFORE SURGERY, the chaplain spends time with the patient and his family. During surgery, the chaplain often stays with the family. After surgery, the chaplain may call in the Recovery Room and then go back to the family.

After surgery, the surgeon tells the family how the surgery went, and that's reassuring.

The chaplain can often say, "I spoke to your wife, and she answered me." That provides a different kind of reassurance.

Working with surgeons isn't always easy.

They're angry men. Dr. Karl A. Menninger wrote in one of his papers that surgeons are men who have found a constructive outlet for their hostility.

They're show-offs. I once knew an eye surgeon who would pile up thirty-five squares of toilet paper and ask you to call out a number from five to thirty. If you yelled out "fourteen," he would take his little knife and promptly, surely, cut through fourteen of those thirty-five pieces of toilet paper.

They are great believers in status. On the *medical* service the word was: "Call Dan Adler—the chief of medicine—any time you think you need to." On the *surgical* service: "Never call Fred Brenner—the chief surgeon—unless you've worked your way up through the hierarchy of assistant residents, assistant chief resident, chief resident—and you'd better have a fantastically good reason."

The standard saying in surgery at MUH was: "The shit flows down from the top."

On the other hand . . .

Surgeons work hard, long hours.

They command tremendous loyalty from their teams.

When they call the chaplain, they usually know just what they want.

They care a lot, most of them.

From my notes on consultation requests from surgeons:

"Chaplain, this man has about a 50-50 chance in surgery day after tomorrow. But if he goes in calm and trusting, that might change to 60-40. Can you help him calm down?"

"Please call on Mrs. Shaffer. Her husband is up for surgery tomorrow, and she suspects the same thing we all do, that he's inoperable. She's a terribly nervous person. If you can help her, you'll be helping me."

"Please stay away from Mr. Treadwell. If he sees a chaplain, he'll be sure he's going to die. Damn fool, but let's try to keep him alive."

"You pray for the patients, don't you? Well, I've got an eight-hour job tomorrow, and my ulcer's kicking up. How about praying for me?"

"Will you convince Mrs. Machmann that her husband's really going to be all right? Nothing I can say gets through. She was prepared to have him die, and when the surgery went well, she wasn't prepared for that."

"Were you praying for Mr. Schultz? If you were, that's all that pulled him through. Say a little prayer of thanks, will you?"

"Here's a list of my patients for tomorrow. Mention them in chapel service, will you?"

"Something's wrong with my best assistant resident. Will you talk to him and see if you can find out what's up?"

Giuseppe Borgia, despite his ominous name, was an open heart surgeon.

Thirty percent of his patients never made it. That didn't mean he was incompetent. It was what is known as "the state of the art." It was just the risk ratio.

I stood talking with Zena Forbush in the Recovery Room, seeing out of the corner of my eye Giuseppe Borgia—by the way, he was a Presbyterian—standing at the foot of a bed looking intently at a small form.

"Is that Giuseppe's patient?"

"Yes. She's not going to make it. Seven years old."

Dr. Borgia saw me and beckoned.

"Stay here a minute with me, Chaplain."

"Not good?"

"A matter of minutes. We've done all we can."

We waited, watching the child and the monitors. One line on a TV set wiggled, leaped, twisted, and finally flattened.

"She's gone."

Tears streamed down Dr. Borgia's face. I knew his colitis would kick up. Too hesitantly, I put my arm around his shoulders. We stood there for a full five minutes, watching the now quiet form. One last look at the monitors.

We die in living color on the TV.

"I'll go talk with the family, Chaplain. By myself. But you be ready. When I come out, you go in."

"You need a kleenex, Joe."

"Yeah. Damn."

MUH trained many foreign surgeons. One of the best—and most nervous—was Farid Attaoullah, a Turk of Lebanese extraction. His specialty was neurosurgery, and he was a delicate master of everything a surgeon needed, except the English language.

"Choplayn Pairkeenz, will you come weeta me to tallek to Meezeez Glook? I 'fraid I not underston wiz hair."

Mrs. Gluck's husband, Ned, had been in a five-car accident and had suffered severe shoulder, neck, and skull damage. Farid had worked on Mr. Gluck for seven hours. He managed to tell me that Mr. Gluck had done very well in surgery, but because

Farid had had to poke, prod, pry, and twist the tissues of poor Mr. Gluck's neck, it was still in tremendously painful condition. Mr. Gluck could swallow only liquids, and those with difficuty. This was what Attaoullah was going to try to tell Mrs. Gluck.

But his first sentence to Nell Gluck did him in.

"Meezeez Glook, your hosband die-et."

And Mrs. Gluck dropped to the floor in a dead faint.

It took me a half hour to get through to her that Farid Attaoullah had been trying to tell her about her husband's liquid diet.

But then, I still can't pronounce Attaoullah.

Few experiences will puzzle or infuriate a surgeon more than the experience of surgery well performed and properly curative which then does not cure. The well-cared-for patient who will not improve is so irritating that the surgeon will quickly label him a "crock," that angry word that precedes referral to chaplains and psychiatrists.

John McGillicuddy had amputated Nathan Carstain's leg after Mr. Carstain had been involved in an industrial accident. I suppose I should say that Dr. McGillicuddy had amputated Mr. Carstain's foot. The amputation was just above the ankle, which had been badly crushed. That was three months before John asked me to see Mr. Carstain, who was back for another amputation, this time just below the knee. John already feared that still a third amputation above the knee would be necessary. Mr. Carstain just wouldn't heal. Diabetes—which often contributes heavily to such problems—had already been ruled out.

In a cool, cheerful room, of which two walls had been decorated from floor to ceiling with cards from friends, Mr. Carstain sat up in his bed bubbling with apparent good humor.

"Mr. Carstain? I'm Chaplain Perkins."

"Come in, come in. Glad to see you. You a Methodist?"

"Nope. Reformed Church."

"What's that? Kind of like Presbyterians?"

"That's right."

"What's the difference?"

"Well, I guess you could say that the Presbyterians are Calvinists from Scotland, and we're Calvinists from Holland."

"Perkins don't sound like a Dutch name to me."

"My mother's name was van den Heuvel."

"Do I know any famous Reformed preachers?"

"Well, you might have heard of Norman Vincent Peale." (*Good grief, he's making sure we don't get to anything important!*)

"Oh, sure. But he don't sound Dutch either."

"Dr. Peale's family was originally Methodist, I think. Mr. Carstain, I hear tell you've got some trouble."

"Aw, no. Doctor Mac's just gonna have to take off a few more inches from this crazy leg of mine."

"Crazy leg?"

"Yep. She won't heal. No good to me anyhow. Can't walk on her."

"She? Her? You make it sound like a person."

"Yeah, I do, don't I? Well, she and me've been pretty involved with each other since the accident. But she's no good to me now. Can't walk on her." (*He's said it twice. Follow it up.*)

"You can't use the leg at all?"

"Well, Doctor Mac, he says I *should* have been able to use the leg with that artificial foot they made me. But I just couldn't put any pressure on her. Hurt a lot."

"So you've tried using the leg, but it hasn't worked."

"No good to me now."

"I'm wondering if you're mad at your leg."

His face changed sharply.

"Damn right I am. Fool thing got herself into trouble. I moved back from that falling block of concrete, and she didn't come with me. Serves her right, don't you think?"

By the time he'd finished, the cheerful mask was back in place, but I'd seen fury. And I thought I'd seen what Nathan Carstain was doing. He was disconnecting himself from the leg, blaming the leg, and letting it—pardon me, "her"—be punished for his slowness in getting out of the way. I was about to say something, but he went on.

"Yep, serves her right. I guess the Lord's punishing that ol' leg."

"The Lord?"

"Sure. Oh, I know you preacher Johnnies don't believe in punishment anymore, but I do. My pastor came in from Severance City the other day. That's where I live. He told me God don't punish, but I know better."

"An eye for an eye and a tooth for a tooth?"

"Hey, you got it! That's right."

". . . and a leg for a leg?" (*I'll never know why I said it.*)

The face changed again. The cheerful mask dropped, and intense suspicion showed.

"Whatcha mean?"

"Well, I guess I was just extending the idea." (*Why is he so suspicious? Fleeting thought: Did he cause somebody to lose a leg?*)

"Well, I just figure the Lord's punishing her for letting me down."

"But, y'know, Mr. Carstain, it seems to me that you're the one that's being punished."

"Eh?"

"It's you whose leg is hurting, it's you who can't walk." (*Don't let him disconnect the leg from himself.*)

"Oh, but I will. After this next amputation, I'll be able to walk on her again."

"So you're kind of looking forward to the operation?"

"Damn tootin' I am. Gonna fix me up."

"And you'll walk on it again then."

"Sure. Once it's fixed up to here."

And he put his hand halfway up his thigh.

"Oh. Is that where Dr. McGillicuddy is going to take it off?"

"Yep. I mean, nope."

And the hand moved down below the knee.

And I decided to try to move in on what I'd seen.

"Mr. Carstain, those industrial accidents are rough, aren't they?"

"Yep. Y'never know what's gonna happen. Why, I seen a man get killed right while he was talkin' to me."

"What happened?"

"Girder fell and pinned him. Cut his leg right off and he bled to death before anybody could stop it."

"Before *you* could stop it?"

"Yes. He was standing talking with me and that girder fell and got him. I saw the blood spurting from his leg and I tried to find the proper pressure point." (By now Nathan Carstain's speech was careful, precise. He was almost reciting.) "I had had the training in Red Cross, you see, and I thought I should find the artery in his leg. They told me later that I should have found the abdominal aorta before it split into the iliac arteries and pressed against his pelvis. But I didn't know that. The amputation was too high up his thing."

I heard the "Freudian slip" but decided not to comment. It turned out later that his friend's genitals had been crushed by the girder.

"Mr. Carstain, that must have been a terrible experience for you." (*You understand it now, Perkins, but how do you get him to see it? Or do you try to get him to see it? He's giving you some signs that he wants to talk about the accident. But will it really help to bring it all up? How shaken will he be? Do you have the skill to pace it properly? Should a psychiatrist take it from here? Are you really right? Does he want to lose the leg to "pay" for his failure to save his friend?*)

"Well, it was pretty bad, but that was a long time ago."

"You'd rather forget it."

"I *had* forgotten it until I had my own accident."

"Brought a lot of it back, didn't it?"

"Sure did. Say, did you say Dr. Peale was originally a Methodist? I'm a Methodist, you know."

And, for the moment, I had my answer. Would it make sense to John McGillicuddy?

It did. Dr. McGillicuddy did the amputation and called for

a series of psychiatric interviews during Mr. Carstain's recovery period.

I never found out whether a third amputation was necessary.

Recovery rooms, providing intensive post-surgical care, have reduced post-surgical mortality tremendously. Zena Forbush, the charge nurse in the RR, presided over a tightly organized madhouse. To an insider, the RR is a cheerful, hopeful, hard-working arena, with careful organization despite a dozen little emergencies every hour. To an outsider, seeing all the bottles and tubes of the life-support systems, the running to and fro, and the patients whose faces are the color of unbaked pie dough, it's a frightening, confusing place. Still, families sometimes try to insist on seeing patients in the RR. At MUH, the RR was hidden around a corner from the surgical suites. But occasionally someone found it. That often meant a call for me.

I was on one of my infrequent "happy calls" in obstetrics, in the middle of a celebration prayer with a delighted young couple who'd had their first child the day before. They were holding hands.

"Chaplain Perkins, Chaplain Samuel Perkins."

"Is that your page, Chaplain?"

" 'Fraid it is. Well, I wish you lots of joy in little Eddie."

"Glad you put that stuff about work in the prayer, Chaplain. It was a good reminder."

"Sure. See you folks."

Dial zero.

"Chaplain Perkins."

"Call the Recovery Room, 2121."

"Chaplain Perkins here."

"Oh, this is Zena Forbush. We've got a crazy man up here. Can you come up?"

"On the double."

The Recovery Room looked its usual madhouse self. No crazy men in sight.

"Hi, Mrs. Forbush. Where's your crazy man?"

"Out on the roof."

"WHAT!"

"Oh, Chaplain, it's half funny and half terrible. See that teen-ager over there? She had an abdominal tumor that Dr. Tanqueray took out this morning. Benign. But her uncle somehow found his way up here and wanted to see her. We didn't let him in, but he caught sight of her through the door, and, well, you know how she looks; not nearly as good as she really is. He'd had something to drink, I think. Anyway, he just went out of his tree, danced around out in the hall like a crazy man, screaming that she was going to die. That's when I called you. Meanwhile, he walked down the hall, out through the door, and out onto the roof of the next building. What'll we do?"

"Well, I guess I'll go out there and find out."

I stepped out through the screen door into the boiling summer heat on top of the laboratory building that butted up against the clinical building. The tar squished under my feet. Fifty feet away, sitting on the edge of the parapet with his feet dangling over, was a red-faced little man jerking his arms in agitation. I'd forgotten to get his name, but maybe Mrs. Forbush didn't even know it.

I stopped ten feet from the man.

"Hello, there."

"WHO ARE YOU?" he screamed.

"I'm the Chaplain."

"Oh, I'm so glad to see you. It's terrible, just terrible."

"You're really upset, aren't you?" I said and was horrified to see him get to his feet on the three-foot-high wall, teetering back and forth.

"Oh, Chaplain, I'm so anxious I don't know if I can stand it."

And then my unconscious did me in.

"Feel pretty jumpy, eh?"

He fell.

Backward.

Onto the roof.

When I had spanned that ten feet—which somehow had grown to a hundred feet in my mind—he was doubled up with laughter.

"Jumpy. Jumpy! Jesus, that's funny!"

He was drunker than a Welsh coal miner on the night before chapel.

One spring Saturday, at eleven o'clock, the Emergency Room called. It had been raining, and I had to drive carefully over the oil-and-water-filmed streets.

Out in Washington Corners, thirty miles northwest, a boy on a motorcycle had lost control and smashed his unhelmeted head against a metal pole. The neurosurgeons were working on his head.

His parents were in the waiting room blaming each other for the accident.

"I told you, George, never to let Denny out of the house without his helmet."

"Madge, dammit, I can't watch the boy every minute."

"You just don't care! If he dies, it's your fault."

"You were the one that insisted I should let him have the cycle."

I decided to ask them to tell me what had happened. Gradually, we pieced the story together. Nobody had seen Denny leave the house. He had consistently refused to wear his helmet unless forced to do so. Apparently, he'd sneaked out of the house so that he wouldn't have to wear the helmet, and both parents knew it.

They were really angry with the boy.

But how can you be angry with a seventeen-year-old boy who may be dying? You turn your anger elsewhere, like a dam diverting a stream. Psychologists call it displacement.

I worked to help the parents calm down. By the time they were a little calmer, Farid Attaoullah was on the scene. His English had improved. He told them that Denny's condition was precarious, that he'd be admitted to the hospital.

For a while, I lost touch with Denny Edmonds and his folks. But one day almost a month later, on Men's Surgery, I saw Mrs. Edmonds in the hall.

"Chaplain Perkins, isn't it?"

"Yes, and you're Denny Edmonds' mother?"

"Yessir. Will you come in and see Denny? He won't talk to us. Maybe he'll talk to you."

I went into the four-bed room. There lay Denny Edmonds with life-support systems hooked up to him. They were breathing for him, feeding him, draining his bladder. Denny would not talk to me either.

He could not.

His brain was so damaged that he couldn't talk to anyone.

I spoke a little with Mrs. Edmonds, prayed with her.

Later I talked with Shelby Cassell, the surgical resident who was covering that floor.

"Shelby, I've just seen Denny Edmonds. I was in the ER when he was brought in. What're things like?"

"Hell, Sam, he's essentially decerebrate.*"

"You seem angry, Shel."

"I fucking well am. Pardon my language. I know you're a chaplain."

"I've heard worse. What're you mad about?"

"That revolving S.O.B. Brady, who had this service last month, hooked the kid up to the Bird and won't unhook him. The kid's dead, Sam. You've heard of death warmed over. Well, that's it right there."**

---

* Decerebrate. The cerebrum is the large portion of the brain with which we do our thinking. To lose the function of that part of the brain is to become decerebrate. Other parts of the brain that work more automatically and control breathing and heartbeat may continue to function. The decerebrate person is often called by that horrible word "vegetable."

** A Bird is an automatic device that controls respiration. To tide a patient over a time when his breathing is irregular, the physician may attach this or some other automatic respiratory-control device to the patient. When the patient can breathe on his own, the device is removed. But sometimes a respirator may be applied to a patient who, everybody knows, will not breathe on his own ever again. Most physicians think that

"Well, your hands are tied, aren't they? No wonder you're mad."

"You know Brady. He blithely put the damn respirator on, knowing he'd be off the service before we knew whether the kid would make it or not. Now he won't take the rest of the responsibility. Chaplain, let me ask you: Is it right to play God like that?"

"Man, that's a rough question, Shel. You guys have to ask it all the time, don't you?"

"Well, I guess we take it on when we go into medicine. That's what you said in that medical ethics symposium last fall."

"Well, Shel, would you want to change the rule?"

"I don't know. I'd hate to take the Edmonds kid off the respirator, but if I had the authority, I think I'd do it. There's only one loose respirator available today. Suppose we needed that Bird for someone else, somebody we could save with it. No, I think it's a good rule. You take the risk of putting somebody on the Bird, you ought to have the conn when it comes to taking him off it. But Brady's copping out."

"You agree, then, that a guy who starts something has a responsibility to finish it if he can?"

"Sure. I can't fight that. I've made that tough decision be-

---

that is irresponsible medicine. The toughest decision, however, is whether to place a respirator on a patient who may breathe on his own again, or may not. You take that risk, and then if the patient goes downhill and is alive only by virtue of such life-support systems, someone must sooner or later disconnect the breathing apparatus, at which point the patient dies.

At MUH, as in some other hospitals I know of, the senior staff has decided that a tremendous amount of thought must be given to a case before taking the huge responsibility of hooking a respirator to a borderline patient. For that reason, they have established the rule that the only physician who may order a respirator removed from a patient is the physician who ordered it connected in the first place. Only Dr. Brady had the authority to remove the respirator from Denny Edmonds. He would not do it. The surgical resident who had the responsibility for the rest of Denny's care, Dr. Shelby Cassell, could only argue; he could not act.

By the way, I later discovered that a "revolving S.O.B." is a man who is an S.O.B. no matter from which angle you look at him.

fore now. I made it as an intern. I was wrong to start the respirator in the first place, and I caught hell for it. But even though my judgment was wrong, I took my lumps, and I'll make a bold decision again tomorrow if I have to, even if I'm wrong. Goddam it, Chaplain, that's what surgery is. You cop out, and you crump out, and you're not a surgeon. Is that playing God?"

"I don't think so. Men have always had to use their skills as stewards."

"Stewards?"

"I see doctors and chaplains and lots of other people as custodians of the talents God gave them. You make a decision like that prayerfully, even if you don't start the prayer by muttering 'Our Father. . . .' You aren't playing God. You're not taking on a part in a play, even if you are in some sense God's hands and feet."

"Where'd you get that idea?"

"From the Bible."

"Well, whoever said it, I agree with them. Does the Bible say anything about copping out?"

"Lots. But not in those words."

"Well, meanwhile, back at the ranch, what do we do about Denny Edmonds?"

"No, not 'what do we do?' At least, I don't think so. The question I see is: What does Shelby Cassell do? I think you know what you can't do. What you can do is put as much pressure on Brady as you can, and maybe go with Brady to the Chief Resident."

"Well, I guess you're right. And I guess I knew that all along. But it helps to bitch about it to you."

"My pleasure. My privilege."

"I wouldn't have your job, listening to people like me bitch all day."

"I don't think I'd have yours either, Shel."

"Who would?"

VII
PSYCHIATRY

PSYCHIATRISTS ARE ATHEISTS.
Psychiatrists are very religious men.
Psychiatrists are crazy.
Psychiatrists are the only ones who are sane.
Psychiatrists are too interested in sex.
Nonsense. Myth. Bosh.

Psychiatrists are ordinary human beings. Some are indeed atheists. But some are Methodist lay leaders, Presbyterian ruling elders, or Episcopal vestrymen. Some are even priests or nuns. Some are mentally ill themselves, some are addicts, some are quite healthy, ordinary human beings. Psychiatrists are indeed quite interested in sex, but for the same reasons you and I are.

We have a hard time thinking of psychiatrists as ordinary people because we want them to have magical powers to heal the mind, or we're afraid they have magical powers to see through us; or both.

There is one odd problem that many psychiatrists do have: dealing with the patient's religious beliefs and thoughts. And it doesn't matter whether the psychiatrist himself is a religious man. He still has a hard time dealing with the religious thoughts of his patients. He is tempted to treat them as part of the patient's problem. He is tempted to reinforce some of them if it will help keep the patient well longer. But most of all, he is tempted to pretend that they don't exist and don't need to be dealt with.

Sometimes he calls the chaplain.

"Chaplain, do you know Miss Tophio?"

It's Ivan Kropp, a first-year resident in psychiatry.

"No, I don't think I do."

"O.K., never mind."

"Wait a minute. Why did you ask?"

"Well, I don't suppose you can do anything about her. But Dr. Bothwell said to ask you."

Terence Bothwell is the Chief of the Psychiatric Service.

"Dr. Kropp, I think you have a hard time believing that I might help."

"Well, frankly, I do. But it *is* a religious problem. At least, her religious behavior is very strange."

"Why not tell me about it?"

"Well, she's a Unitarian, I think. She got hold of a Bible the other day—I don't know how—and since then she's been quoting Scripture even though we took the Bible away, of course."

(It's common practice in most mental hospitals and psychiatric wards in general hospitals to forbid patients to have Bibles. The staff often feels that Bibles disturb the patients. The same staff often permits the same patients to see highly disturbing movies.)

"And what is it you wonder, Doctor?"

"Well, we don't understand why a Unitarian would be interested in the Bible in the first place. And why does she now quote Scripture so much?"

"Well, first of all, what Scripture does she quote?"

"I don't know. Just Scripture. Different things."

"Dr. Kropp, if a patient started hallucinating and trying to tell you what he saw in his hallucinations, would you pay attention to what he thought he was seeing?"

"Of course!"

"Well, to begin with, then, I'd suggest that you pay a similar kind of attention to what Miss Tophio is saying when she quotes Scripture. What she says may turn out to be a key to what's going on for her."

"I hadn't thought of that."

"How active a Unitarian is she? What's her connection with her church?"

"I don't know. Just a Unitarian. That's all it said in the chart."

"Well, why don't we get a religious history?"

"What's that?"

"You take social histories, marital histories, physical histories, histories of everything else about the patient's past. But few psychiatrists ever take a religious history."

"Would that be relevant?"

"In many cases it would be, and I think it might be particularly interesting and relevant in the case of a patient who displays behavior that appears to be religious in nature."

"That sounds like a good idea. But what would you ask?"

"Well, perhaps we could talk with Miss Tophio together, and then afterward you and I could talk about it."

"O.K. How about one o'clock tomorrow?"

"Fine."

After the conversation with Ivan Kropp, a few reflections. I'd trapped myself. While I was talking with him, I could pretend that it was a kind of teaching dialogue. But now I realized that I had been essentially putting him down. What do you want, Perkins? Do you want to shake up an arrogant, insensitive know-it-all? You may have done a good job of that by being a know-it-all yourself. You forgot that he may already be scared by the strange behavior of his patient—strange to him, anyhow.

Or did you want to help Kropp learn something new, become a more sensitive, better-rounded psychiatrist? What you just did, didn't help much.

But he *was* willing at least to learn something in the long run. You've got a chance to help him see something. If you can be a better teacher, maybe he can be a better healer. Try for a conversation with him both before and after you see Miss Tophio. See what he does know about the patient. Let him help you help him. Pay the same kind of attention to him that you want him to pay to the patient.

So the next day I had lunch with him before we went to see Miss Tophio.

"It's a funny thing, Chaplain."

"What's that?"

"I'd never considered doing a religious history. And it's not that I'm not a religious man myself. In fact, I'm a Catholic convert, and very active in St. Bede's parish."

"Yeh. Well, it really *is* a funny thing, but you're not alone. Psychiatrists really don't seem to feel easy about touching religious issues with their patients."

"How do you explain that?"

"I don't have much of an explanation. There seem to be different reasons. Sometimes I find myself thinking that people see us as a rival group of magicians, and we somehow buy into that."

"Could be. But tell me, just what do you look for in a religious history? What are you after?"

"Essentially, I think you're after a number of things. What are the patient's stated religious beliefs? Is he having trouble with any of them? Maybe one of the most important questions is: How is the patient *using* his religion? Or, what *kind* of God does he seem to believe in? And underneath, you're always asking: Does all this have any relation to his illness? In fact, you have some information that I'd like you to share with me if you will. Mainly this: How do you see Miss Tophio's illness?"

"Well, it isn't easy. She's thirty-two and lives alone in an apartment on the second floor of an old house. Teaches art at

Grand Centre High School. Her landlady lives alone down-stairs—an elderly widow. The landlady went up to collect the rent and found the patient all scrunched up and naked on the floor with her eyes wide open and staring. Thought she was dead, then saw her move. Called her doctor, who wouldn't touch it with a ten-foot pole. Then called her pastor; she be-longs to The Methodist Church. I think his name is Gross-kreutz."

"Jim Grosskreutz, yeah. I had him here as a student."

"Oh, yeah? Well, he saw that it was a psychiatric case, got the old lady to help him bundle Miss Tophio up, and brought her to the Emergency Room. They admitted her right away."

"What happened then?"

"Just about nothing. No trouble keeping clothes on her since admission. But she hadn't said word one since she came in, un-til that damn Bible showed up. By the way, we have no idea how she got it."

"Will she talk with you?"

"Yes. Just says she has to be open to the Spirit. What does that mean, do you know?"

"It could mean several things, but I can't really guess. Why don't we go see her?"

"Good."

Small, bare room. Neatly made bed. One comfortable chair by a barred window. The window is barred inside and out. Miss Tophio can't get to any glass. (The hospital jargon is: Keep the patient away from "sharps," meaning anything either sharp in itself or breakable into sharp-edged pieces. Also: no belts or anything else the patient could use to hang herself. Routine for all patients, whether you think they're suicidal or not.)

The door stands open, but Kropp knocks on the doorjamb anyway. (Observe the boundaries, something to which psy-chiatrists tend to be more sensitive than do other physicians.)

"Gretel, may we come in?"

She just looks back, gives no signals. Kropp and I sit side by side on the bed. It's not the thing to do, but there are no other chairs.

Kropp again. "Gretel, this is Chaplain Perkins. He'd like to talk with you."

Her eyes brighten, get dull again. My turn.

"Miss Tophio, would you be willing to talk with me a while?"

"Yes." No emotion in the voice.

Already the relays are clicking in my head. The flat, emotionless voice says: schizophrenic process. (*Danger: if you start diagnosing, you won't hear.*)

"Dr. Kropp says that you're a Unitarian."

"That's right."

Pause.

She goes on.

"I don't think I'll be a Unitarian anymore."

"No more?"

"Some Unitarians believe in God. Some don't. They don't. I do."

"It sounds as though you've been doing some thinking about God."

"Yes."

"Can you tell me about that? What are your thoughts?" (*Too invasive! You're moving too fast. Will she answer?*)

"God is Light. Eternal Light. I want to move toward the Light."

"Light. Some people think of God as a person, but you say light. Is there a difference?"

"Yes. God is not a person. God is Light. Dr. Kropp is in the light. Please move, Dr. Kropp."

He looks at me, moves over, and the light from the window falls on Gretel Tophio.

"You want the light to shine on you?"

"Perhaps you are understanding something."

"Perhaps, but not as much as I'd like to."

"I want to be enlightened."

Odd thought. She sounds more like a Zen Buddhist. Use the thought.

"How will you achieve enlightenment?"

"By being open."

"Miss Tophio, when your landlady found you, she told us you were scrunched up on the floor of your apartment, naked."

"Not scrunched. Spread-eagled."

"And your eyes were wide open."

"Yes."

"You were opening yourself to the light, weren't you?"

"Perhaps you are understanding something."

"I wonder if you think you can tell me anything about your pilgrimage."

And at this point everything changes. Her eyes light up, her body becomes a little more tense. Her voice takes on color. A moment ago she had to be crazy; now she does not. I wonder if Kropp notices.

"My parents were Unitarians, you know. (*I don't know, and perhaps I should stop her right there, but I don't.*) They talked a lot about philosophy and religion. But their lives were all tight."

"Perhaps your life was too."

"Well, that's the point, isn't it? I was all closed up. Closed off. I knew that that was not right for me. I have been searching. They said God was freedom, but I felt no freedom. Talk, talk, talk—that's all it was. They didn't experience freedom. I didn't either. I had no friends. I knew no love. I looked for light. I found it."

"Do you know how it happened?"

"Pentecostal fire."

"H'm?"

"Pentecostal fire. I went to Pentecostal meetings. They had fire. They had light. They were open. Part of the time, anyway. Now I have my own fire and light."

"How did that happen?"

"*You* know." (*And now she is suddenly crazy again. The light in her eyes goes out; she slumps.*)

"You think I know?"

"*You* know."

I play a hunch.

"God is love as well as light?"

"See. You know."

Damn! I played a hunch. The hunch was right. Playing it was wrong. I brought into her feelings that I had magic. How do I get out of this?

"Perhaps I am understanding something. But I am not understanding as much as you think I am."

"Love and light are the same. I found love. *You* know."

"I do not answer.

"*You* know. I found love. Are you understanding something?"

"Miss Tophio, a minute ago you said you knew no love. I think perhaps you were telling us that you knew no lover. But now you know a lover. Is that what you are saying?" (*And I mean the old Biblical use of the word "know." And she understands it.*)

"Yes. A man. Not a man. A man."

Now it is time to try a risky understanding of what she is struggling with.

"Miss Tophio. You have had a lover. He is a man. But you are afraid to love a man. It is safer to love God, to love Light." (*And I do not say the rest: that she was having intercourse with the Light when the landlady found her.*)

"You are understanding something."

Anton Boisen, the pioneer in education of ministers in mental hospitals, insisted that a psychotic episode can be understood as an attempt to solve a religious struggle, or a moral one. After thirty-two years of closed-up virginity, Gretel Tophio had known a man. Was it right? Was it wrong? She couldn't decide. One way out: Focus on God as your lover.

I was understanding something. But it was not the only way to understand Miss Tophio.

Dr. Ivan Kropp was also understanding something. It excited him so much that he could not wait to talk about it. When an aide came in to ask Miss Tophio to go to OT (Occupational Therapy), we talked.

"That's it! You had the key! How did you know?"

"I didn't *know*, Dr. Kropp. I don't have magic either. It's just that paying attention to the meaning of religious language is *one* of the keys to understanding. You might well have gotten to the same point by carefully investigating her relationships with her parents."

"Well, what should I do now?"

"That's hard to say. I don't really want to direct you. All I'd say is that now you're in a position to add something to your work with Miss Tophio. Just one thing . . ."

"What's that?"

"I think that if you call her Gretel, you're speaking to the childish side of her. Why not call her by her adult name: Miss Tophio?"

Telling this next story will be hard. It's going to seem as if I'm hiding something from you; and I am. But I think you'll see why.

Teri Williams, the charge nurse on Men's Medicine, was responding to my questions about troubled patients. As we stood by the chart rack, up ran Dawn Foster, a student nurse.

"Mrs. Williams! Mrs. Williams!"

Her face was working. You couldn't tell if she was about to cry or to vomit.

"Miss Foster, we can't run in the halls." (*Was Teri just being prim and proper, or was she lowering the stakes for Miss Foster a little?*)

"Yes, Mrs. Williams. I'm sorry, but it was just so awful . . ."

"What was awful, Miss Foster?"

"Mr. Corrigan . . ."

And here's where I hide something temporarily. Dawn Foster told her story about Mr. Corrigan, and you'll have to wait for a while to hear that story.

What she said sounded to me like a good case for the seminar I attended for psychiatric residents. It was typical of the kind of thing that happens often in a general hospital. But it was also the kind of thing that nursing and medical staffs have a hard time understanding.

I presented it to the group like a detective story.

"Mr. C. is a patient on Men's Medicine. He is fifty-nine. Because of his illness, he has lost his job. He probably won't get another. During his hospitalization, he has had a number of quarrels with his wife and thinks she is about to leave him. Currently, his legs are paralyzed, and they may remain so. His hospital regimen calls for him to remain flat on his back. That is hard since he was a very active man until his current illness, which came on suddenly. He cannot move on his own. He is very depressed. When the student nurse comes to see him, however, he becomes very talkative. He finds it difficult to let her care for the other patients in the room.

"Two days ago, Miss Foster was talking with him and made as if to leave. It bothered him very much, and he wanted to make her stay with him and pay attention to him."

"What did he do?"

The people around the table looked puzzled, with one exception. The only person who looked as if he knew what happened was a senior psychiatrist. But the rest seemed to think I had left something out. I went around the table, skipping Dr. Mackintosh, the senior man.

"I don't know."

"Aren't there any other facts, Chaplain?"

"Nope."

Mackintosh grinned: "You don't need any other facts."

"I can't guess."

"Search me."

And so on.

"Dr. Mackintosh?"

"He exposed himself, of course."

The room was full of questions.

"What do you mean?"

"How do you know?"

"Aren't you guessing?"

"Well," from a resident, "how in the world *did* you know?"

"The man is paralyzed. He has very little available to him. His wife is angry with him. He has lost his job. All the things that spell maleness have been taken away from him. He needed to do something dramatic to hold on to Miss Foster, here. What else did he have left?"

"But the sight of his genitals drove Miss Foster away!"

"And then what happened?" I asked.

No one spoke.

"Well, Miss Foster ran down to the nurses' station and told Mrs. Williams and me what had happened. And Mrs. Williams charged down and scolded Mr. C."

"How long a time did she spend with him?"

"Oh, about fifteen minutes. And then she brought the student back and had him apologize to her."

"So he got a lot of attention?"

"I guess you could say that."

"In fact," finished the psychiatrist, "our Mr. C. got just about what he wanted."

"Attention?"

"That and more. He got a reaction to what little maleness he had left."

The seminar provided useful case study. But it did more than that. It also bridged the gap that usually exists between psychiatrists and the rest of the staff.

Other doctors have a hard time using psychiatrists. They seldom guess that the psychiatrist may help to explain a patient's unusual behavior. They think of self-exposure and other behavior problems as bad, troublesome, immoral. They seldom think that the behavior is caused by something happening to the patient. With his belief that all behavior has meaning, the psychiatrist can—if asked in the right way—make clear the meaning of some problems.

He can also help the staff understand what to do about such problems.

A different student nurse was assigned to Mr. Corrigan, with instructions to talk with him as much as possible. He never exposed himself again. He also regained some of his self-confidence.

I never did call on him.

Some psychiatrists don't have so much difficulty in dealing with the religious ideas of patients. Bill Hart didn't. He was MUH's Chief Resident in Psychiatry one year, and a personal friend. Everything you think a doctor should be, Bill was— warm, tender, tough, salty, able to make tough decisions.

We often had lunch together.

"Hey, Bill."

"Sam! Pull up a loose stool and siddown."

"How are you?"

"Tolerable. How's chaplaining?"

"Heavy."

"Say, Sam, I had something I wanted to kick around with you."

"Shoot, buddy."

"I've got a patient who's a minister. Rather not tell you who he is, but sure would like to ask you about him."

"O.K."

"Well, he's having trouble with his wife, and that's why he's coming in. Lackanooky."

"What?"

"No sex life."

"I've heard of it."

"But he never wants to discuss his problems. Always brings up counseling cases instead, wants me to help him figure out what to do with his parishioners."

"You understand that, don't you, Bill?"

"Aw, sure. It's resistance to treatment. But at the same time, he really does have some tough counseling cases of his own. They're interesting. Matter of fact, he's not a bad counselor. But it sure beats the shit out of treatment."

"Bill, I think I hear a proposition coming."

"You betcha my foot you do. How about if I refer him to you for consultation on his counseling cases? That would clear up my treatment problem with him."

"Think it really would?"

"Well, not exactly. But if I could get the consultation stuff off my back, then it'd be easier to deal with his resistance as resistance. Now if you're willing, I'll tell you who he is, and we can go to work on it."

"Bill, I could see him once every two weeks."

"That's good enough. Do you know Garrett Groton?"

"Rector of All Saints' Episcopal."

"That's the guy."

"Sure, I know him. How do you want to work it?"

"Well, I'll refer him to you, and he can call you. You take it from there."

What happened, of course, was that I did take Father Groton on in consultation. But he still kept bringing the same cases to Bill. When Bill called it resistance, Garrett Groton said I wasn't helping him, but Bill steadfastly turned it down. Meanwhile, Groton started talking with *me* about his sexual difficulties with his wife.

Resistance is a powerful thing. You want help, and you *don't* want it. You want to change, but the way of life you have is what's comfortable. It's all you've ever known. So you go to a psychiatrist for therapy, and to a chaplain for consultation about your work. Then you try to turn the consultation into therapy and the therapy into consultation.

Finally, we both saw Garrett Groton together in Bill's office.

"Father Groton, Chaplain Perkins and I think that we need to clear things up with you. This is by way of an announcement, I guess. You know that you are talking about therapy things with him, and about counseling cases with me, and it must be the other way around."

"But I'm not aware that I'm doing it!"

"Now you are. And we've decided to keep you aware. Sam?"

"Yes. Gary, I'm not going to listen to your problems with your wife any more. When you bring them up, I'm simply going to say that you need to take that up with Dr. Hart."

"And if you bring up counseling cases with me, I'm simply going to say that you need to take that up with Chaplain Perkins. And that's all either of us is going to say."

The following week, Garrett Groton was fifteen minutes late for his appointment. He had a good excuse, but I knew it was an excuse—that he was mad at Bill Hart and at me. (I found out later that he'd been twenty minutes late for his therapy hour with Bill.) He tried "crossing the wires" with me, and I said what Bill and I had agreed we'd say.

"Gary, I won't discuss Nancy with you. That's for your hour with Dr. Hart."

"I didn't realize I was doing it."

"You're doing it. Stop it."

"You bastard!"

"Now about Mrs. Anderson . . ."

"Well, she came in on time and was dressed as usual . . ."

And Father Groton finally went to work.

VIII
DEATH

MAYBE I'VE ALREADY DEALT with death enough.

Maybe too much to suit most people.

It's often been said that in our day death is replacing sex as the most obscene thing around. If that's true, then you may be offended if I say more about death.

But I have to. When I wrote about death or dying people in earlier chapters, it was mostly about people who happened to die. This chapter is different in one important way: It's about working with people who know they are dying. Like Eloise Hammar.

Eloise had the Bad Disease. A form of cancer called malignant melanoma. One of my psychiatrist friends said that if he had a malignant melanoma on his ankle, he'd make sure the doctor amputated his leg at the hip. Eloise's had started on the side of her neck. When I first saw her, they had just dug as deeply as they could into her neck, and the left side of her face was badly swollen.

Eloise Hammar was eighteen. She'd never be nineteen.

In spite of the swelling, she managed a big grin when I came in. Her mother, seeing the big blue cross hanging from my jacket pocket, frowned as hard as Eloise smiled.

"You're a chaplain, aren't you?" said Eloise.

"That's right. Chaplain Perkins."

"Well, good, I want to—"

"Eloise just had surgery last week, Chaplain. I think she needs her rest."

"Nonsense, Mother, he's just the man I want to see."

Reluctantly, Mrs. Hammar subsided for a moment.

"How *are* you doing, Miss Hammar?"

"She's just fine, Chaplain. The surgery was a real success."

Mrs. Hammar really took over at that point. Brightly chattering and brightly dressed, she twittered like a whole cageful of brightly plumed lovebirds. Eloise was fine. The surgeons were wonderful. The nurses were so helpful. Eloise was going home next week. She'd only have to have a few little treatments.

I watched the big grin fade ever so slowly from Eloise's face. The more her mother talked, the more depressed the girl became. After the depression came anger. I looked for an opening, and finally Mrs. Hammar took a deep breath between paragraphs.

"Eloise, you look distressed."

"I am, Chaplain Perkins."

"Why, dear, whatever is the matter?"

"Mother, will you please leave the room?"

"Of course. We're bothering you, aren't we? Come, Chaplain—"

"No! Mother, will *you* please get out of here. I'm going to die, and I want to talk to this man about it."

"You see, Chaplain, she *is* upset. Let's step outside and—"

"MOTHER! GO! If you don't leave now, I'll tell the nurse not to let you visit me anymore. You have *got* to let me die *my* way."

Mrs. Hammar glanced at me. If looks could kill, *I*'d be dead. Her face fell, became expressionless; she walked out.

"Now, Chaplain, we can talk."

"O.K."

"About dying. Me dying."

"Tell me about it."

"Do you wonder how I know?"

"I guess I do."

"Well, Dr. Trehearne told me. Point-blank."

"He really laid it on the line, didn't he?"

"Yes. At first, I didn't believe him. Not me. What eighteen-year-old can believe that?"

"Maybe at first nobody can."

"How about old people?"

"Not even old people, sometimes."

"Oh. Well, after that I thought of all the people who deserved to die more than me. I even wanted Dr. Trehearne to die. I even dreamed he might catch the cancer from me. That's one of the things I wanted to ask you. Is that bad?"

"You mean unhealthy?"

"No, I mean wicked. Is it wicked to feel like that?"

"Do you really need to have me tell you?"

"I guess not. I decided it wasn't wicked. It's my *death*, and I have to do it my way. Do you read the charts?"

"Sometimes. I've read yours, if that's what you're asking."

"Is there a thing about a physical exam in there?"

"Sure."

"Does it say I'm a virgin?"

"Probably. I didn't notice. Why?"

"Well, I am. And I used to be proud of it."

"Used to be."

"I'd like to have intercourse before I die."

"Can you say more about that?"

"Just that I'd like to have every important experience people can have at least once before I die. I even prayed about it. I said to God that I'd be willing to die if I could just have intercourse first. With an orgasm, of course. You don't look shocked."

"Should I?"

"Well, I'm being pretty frank. What do you think about what I've said?"

"I guess I think that that kind of promise to God isn't too different from the other things you've said."

"Not wicked?"

"Not wicked."

"But dumb."

"H'm?"

"Well, you know, even if the thing I'm thinking isn't wicked to think about, it wouldn't necessarily be wise to do it, would it?"

"I see. It might be a mistake to do it, but you don't think it'd be a mistake to want to."

"I've got my choice. I can die with an orgasm or without one. But the choice I *really* want is the one that lets me go down with my banners flying, and . . ."

"And?"

"I *think* that's staying a virgin. But, gosh, knowing you're going to die soon changes a lot of things."

"You're looking at things in a new way."

"Well, the kind of thing that keeps going through my mind is something like this: I guess I'd be willing to let it happen if . . ."

"If what?"

"If a lot of things. If I could, you know . . ."

"Have intercourse."

"Yes, and lots more. See Paris. Paint a really good picture. Help my mother accept this. You know."

"Help your mother accept your death?"

"Sure. She's still back where I was when I first heard about it from Dr. Trehearne. She won't believe it, won't talk about it, won't let me talk about it. She's convinced herself that it won't happen."

"Do you think that maybe she needs to do all that pretending?"

"I guess she does. But can you imagine what it's going to be like for her when it happens? I'm afraid she's going to be like one of those women whose son was killed in Korea. You know, keep his room just like it was, and everything."

"You want to help her. How could you do it?"

"Well, I've started to think that I have to be blunt with her, almost cruel. I've thought that when I go home next week, I want to start giving away things that I own before I have to come back to the hospital. Another thing I've thought is that maybe it'd be better if I didn't come back to the hospital."

"I'm not sure I understand."

"Well, maybe it'd be better for reality if I died at home."

"I guess I'm wondering if some of what you're saying isn't still some of that anger you talked about—as if you wanted to be a little hard on your mother."

"Maybe, I'm not sure. I know I'm angry with her. I feel that I'm a lot more mature than she is. But I'm also thinking of how I can make it possible for her to go on living after I'm gone."

"A mixture of anger and care."

"Sure. Say, I'm getting tired, and I don't think I can talk much longer. Could you come back tomorrow? I still want to ask you about life after death."

"Yes, I'll be back."

It wasn't until quite a number of years later that Dr. Elizabeth Ross, in her book *On Death and Dying,* put some of what I was seeing in order. Dying patients, Dr. Ross found, go through a series of five stages: denial, anger, bargaining, depression, and finally, acceptance. When I saw Eloise Hammar, she was at the bargaining stage. Back then, it would have been nice to know that next she would become depressed.

But I never saw that stage. I saw Eloise three more times during the following week; after that, she went home. The depression came two months later. When she finally returned to MUH, it was only four days before she died.

Dr. Ross points out that in the final stages of acceptance, a dying person has said his good-bys and often withdraws almost completely from talking with others, even those most close. It wasn't until that happened that Mrs. Hammar was finally able to ask for help. We sat for long hours in the room, each just holding Eloise's hand. The day she died, Eloise turned her head slightly on the pillow and smiled her big smile.

"Chaplain Perkins . . ."

"Yes, Eloise."

"I'm still a virgin."

"That's what you decided, eh?"

"M-h'm. Nobody ever gets everything. But I got to choose and I chose. I did what I chose to do."

"Yes."

"Tell anybody who asks you that that's all that counts."

"I will."

Then she fell asleep. Twenty minutes later she woke again. "Chaplain Perkins, did you ever read *Dandelion Wine*?"

"Yes."

"I like Bradbury."

"So do I."

"Do you remember what great-grandma said?"

"I think I know what you mean: 'There's one last tart I haven't bit on.' "

" 'One tune I haven't whistled.' "

"I remember."

Eloise puckered her lips and blew soundlessly.

"And," as Ray Bradbury put it, "the sea moved her back down the shore."

Dorothy Beasley's dying brought several of us face-to-face with one of the most difficult issues.

I'd first called on Dorothy after her first surgery, which revealed that no surgery could save her. She left the hospital soon after to settle her affairs. Leaving in August, she returned in December. The house physician assigned to her was an intern named Barry Alders.

Leaving Dorothy's room one afternoon, I bumped into Dr. Alders in the doorway. Dorothy called us both in.

"Chaplain, I'm going to ask Dr. Alders some questions, and I want you to listen . . . Dr. Alders, what's in the IV (intravenous) you're giving me?"

Barry Alders had a habit of saying nothing more than he needed to.

"Steroids, mostly."

"Are they keeping me alive?"

"They are for now."

"Are they the stuff that's making my face puff up?"

"Probably."

"If you keep giving me the steroids, how long will they keep me alive?"

"Hard to say. A week, two, three. We don't know."

"If you stopped giving me that medicine, how long would it take me to die?"

"We don't know that either."

"But less than a week?"

"Probably."

"Make your best guess, Doctor."

"O.K. Thirty-six hours."

"It's costing my husband about a hundred dollars a day to keep me here. Not Blue Cross. My husband. Our daughter should go to college next year. I literally can't afford to live. Will you take out the IV?"

"I can't answer that. Not now."

"Chaplain, do you understand what I'm saying?"

"Yes, Mrs. Beasley, I do."

"Well, why won't Dr. Alders answer me?"

"He said he couldn't answer you *now*. Maybe he can later."

"Well, you both know what I want."

She waved her hand in dismissal.

Outside the door.

"Cup of coffee, Barry?"

"There's some in the conference room. Jesus, I've gotta talk to you."

"I thought maybe you did."

We drifted down the hall, dimly lighted by the late afternoon sun. In the conference room, Barry Alders threw himself into a chair.

"Chaplain, I swear I'm gonna do it."

"Do what?"

"Pull the IV."

"That's what she wants, isn't it?"

"Sure. And she's got good reasons. And she's right. And I

told the truth in there. With the steroids going, she's got maybe three weeks, and without them three days at the most—and thirty-six hours is more like it."

"Who's your AR?" (Assistant Resident. Every intern is supervised by an assistant resident whose word is usually law.)

"Bob Schumacher."

"Talked to him about it?"

"Not yet. Do you know him well? What'll he say?"

"I don't have the slightest idea. I do think he'll listen."

"Well, I will then. But what do you think? What's the religious point of view. My church—I'm Catholic—is death on euthanasia."

"Yes, it is. But is what she's asking for euthanasia?"

"I don't know. What do you mean?"

"Well, the Catholic Church's position is that in the face of certain death you do *not* need to use heroic measures to keep a patient alive. But if there's any chance at all—"

"There isn't. I was honest with her."

"Then what you have to decide is whether or not keeping the steroids going is heroics. If it isn't heroics, you've got to keep on treating her. But if keeping up the steroids is heroics, you can stop—from the *Church's* point of view."

"But not around here?"

"Let's find Schumacher and ask."

"He ought to be around in about ten minutes. Let's grab him."

We did.

Bob obviously wished we hadn't asked.

"Oh, Christ, I don't know. What is it you're really asking?"

"Well, the patient's Catholic and so am I. Chaplain Perkins says that stopping the steroids would be O.K. in the Church's eyes. It's what she wants, and I think it makes sense. I want to know about Midbank."

"Midbank, Schmidbank. You want to know what *I* think. Well, I'm with you. But I doubt the hospital will allow it."

"So then don't give me that Midbank-Schmidbank stuff. That's exactly the problem."

"Chaplain, this is your bailiwick. I don't even know what's at stake."

"O.K., give me five minutes. Look, medicine is a kind of religion itself. You may be Catholic, and, Bob, I know you're a Lutheran of sorts, but you're both also doctors, and I think your idea of what medicine asks of you is at stake here.

"The Catholic religion says you do all you can to save lives but when a life is definitely lost, there are limits to what you must do. However that's not what medicine says, at least around here. Death is the enemy. You have to hold him off like Horatius at the bridge. You fight down to the last corpuscle. That's not the Christian point of view, not in any branch of the Christian religion I know of. But medicine has its own dogmas, and this is often one of them.

"Dan Adler's your Chief of Service, and if you want to buck it up to him, you can. You know you'd get a hearing. But you know Dan. His first question would be: 'What do *you* think, Doctor?' So you'd better know what you think."

"Well, Sam, is there a guiding rule? Is there some kind of ethics we can go by from a Christian point of view?"

"Sure. Joseph Fletcher says that love is the 'middle term.' [A technical phrase from philosophical and theological ethics. It refers to a kind of focal point around which all ethical decisions must center.] If it is, then the ethical question becomes something like this: What is the most loving thing to do under the circumstances?"

"I can buy that."

"So can I. I think Fletcher's right. So you take out the needle, you give Mrs. Beasley some analgesic help, she dies in thirty-six hours, and then: Does Mr. Beasley slap MUH with a malpractice suit?"

"Dr. Schumacher, Dr. Robert Schumacher." It was the page.

"Well, we didn't decide anything." Schumacher speaking.

Alders looked hard at both of us and walked out first.

Four days later Mrs. Beasley died.

I saw Alders and asked: "What did you decide?"

"I decided to lie."

"H'm?"

"I decided that I'd pull the IV's myself, but let the record show that I kept them going."

"Big decision."

"Yes, but I couldn't go through with it. I kept the IV's going after all. The truth's pretty important."

"Yep. So what is the truth?"

"The truth is that Mrs. Beasley slipped her own needle. We didn't find out until morning, and we started it again, but the break was enough, I guess. She died in the afternoon."

Question: Did Barry Alders cop out?

It's so much easier when you have absolutes of some kind. If you go by the absolute principle that you fight it all the way down to the line—the medical dogma at MUH—you will at least be comfortable. You can say things such as: we did all we could.

But is it true?

The doctor did all he could to save the life. If that's what you mean, it's true.

But did he do all he could to ease the patient's mind? The answer must be No. Was his action based on care and concern for the whole person Dorothy Beasley was, and not just for her failing body? No.

The dogma says that if a doctor thinks about those things, he will lose his nerve as a doctor. You don't ask about love first. You don't ask about concern first. You don't ask about the patient's peace of mind first. You can only afford to ask those questions if your first question is: Am I keeping her alive?

Not all hospitals follow that dogma. Nor all physicians.

When they do, then they have to decide whether to be physicians first or Christians first. (Or, by the way, good Jews first.) The demands of the two religions are not always the same, and medicine *is* a religion.

The chaplain tries to build a bridge between the two.

Question: Did Perkins cop out?

IX
STUDENTS

SIX FEET SIX INCHES TALL and all joints. Blond. Shy. Nurses told me he was cute.

He had just finished his second year at Mount Tabor Divinity School and was spending twelve weeks at MUH as a student chaplain.

His name was Reginald DeBray. Reggie.

After another year at Mount Tabor he would be ordained as a Methodist minister. The dean at the seminary told me that Reggie was one of the most talented students they had: a fine Bible scholar, a writer of well-constructed papers based on sound research, a preacher of promise.

Yep.

Right now our scholar-paper writer-preacher sat in my office with a hangdog look. His face was flushed, his breathing raspy, every muscle of his body tense, and his face was pulled into a long embarrassed scowl.

Underneath all that, he was angry with me.

We were engaging in a difficult conversation, partly educational, maybe a little therapeutic, and he was hating me for it from head to toe.

I was his supervisor.

Earlier that day I'd started the morning with a brief meeting of my four students: Reggie, Tim Logan (Catholic priest), Larry Sissman (another Mount Tabor student), and Delbert

Donohue (an experienced Methodist pastor on leave for the summer from his congregation).

Each man had an assignment: Reggie to Men's Medicine, Tim to Men's Surgery, Larry to Women's Medicine, and Del to Women's Surgery. Each was attached to the assistant resident in charge of each of the four services. The service they were on would be their base for the whole summer, to provide a "home" for each man. But in addition they would take special assignments.

Tim would respond to any "Dr. Edgar Terman" call by heading for the Emergency Room.

Larry would pick up any special calls that came by telephone into the Chaplain's Office. My secretary would have him paged.

Del would cover Pediatrics in addition to his home base in Women's Surgery.

Reggie would take cases on personal assignment from me. I tried to make them challenging assignments.

I'd sent Reggie to see Edgar Antell, a patient whom I'd known from several previous bouts with cancer. Now Mr. Antell was in the hospital for the last time. He had been tremendously angry with his disease—mad at doctors, mad at God, mad at nurses, mad at me. He had progressed past that point to an acceptance of his coming death at the very end of his previous admission. Now he had come in to die.

Reggie was scheduled for supervision at ten thirty. He'd had time to see Mr. Antell and to write at least a sketchy note about the interview.

But he hadn't done it.

"Well, Reg, how did it go with Mr. Antell?"
"It didn't."
"What do you mean, 'it didn't'?"
"I didn't see him."
"Why not?"
And this is the point at which you first met Reggie, scowling at me. My question, meant as a request for more information, had been heard as the first line of a scolding.

"Well, I don't know why not."

"Think about it. What happened?"

"Well, it started out O.K. I went up to Miss Peabody and introduced myself, said I'd come to see Mr. Antell. She said I'd have to wait a minute because they were giving him some kind of treatment. So I went down and had a cup of coffee. I futzed around for a while and then went back up there, got as far as the door, and went back to ask Miss Peabody some kind of question, got into a discussion of Mr. Antell's illness with her, and then went back to the door. I saw that I only had fifteen minutes in which to see him and figured that wasn't enough time. So here I am."

"You're saying that you found at least three ways to avoid seeing Mr. Antell."

"No, goddam it! I wasn't avoiding seeing him. At first I couldn't see him, and then I realized I didn't know enough about him. I had to check that out, didn't I? And then there wasn't enough time left."

"But you really didn't want to see him."

"How can you say that?"

"Because of the evidence, Reg. We broke up here at eight fifteen. You were scheduled for supervision at ten thirty. You had two hours and fifteen minutes, and one assignment. You didn't do the assignment. Let's talk about why."

"All right! I didn't want to see him. Does that make you feel any better?"

"How does it make you feel?"

"Bad. Shitty. I'm a horse's ass. Right?"

"Wrong. You're a chaplain who wasn't able to complete an assignment. You're a student who expects the instructor to lay him out. Most of all, you're a man who needs to understand what happened."

"Sheesh, Sam, I don't *know* what happened."

"Well, let's go back to the point we've agreed on. You didn't want to see Mr. Antell. Do you have any idea why?"

"Sure I do. He's dying. He may die tonight, this afternoon."

"And?"

"And you sent me into a situation you knew I couldn't handle."

"No. I sent you into a situation you're going to have to deal with for the rest of the summer and the rest of your life."

"Well, I couldn't deal with it today."

"Again you're having trouble dealing with the real issue, Reggie. The real issue is: What is it about a dying man that you don't think you can handle?"

"I won't be able to answer his questions. He's going to ask me why he's dying, what the purpose of it all is, why a man thirty-one years old has to die. *I* don't know the answers."

"You're suggesting that I do know those answers."

"Well, don't you?"

"When did I ever have magic answers?"

"Christ, *I* don't know! Maybe there aren't any answers."

"Maybe there aren't."

"Then what do you do?"

"Why are you so sure Mr. Antell is going to ask questions like that?"

"Well, I would, if I were thirty-one and dying."

"I think that it is in fact you who is asking those questions. You think you have to know before you see Edgar Antell. And you don't know. So you're mad at me, at the doctors, at God."

"Yes, that's right. I am mad at all of you. What's the point of being a minister if you have to cope with stuff like this?"

"Suppose that stuff like this is exactly what you do have to cope with as a minister."

"I can't do it."

"Can't do what?"

"Cope with this dying stuff."

"Well, Mr. Antell didn't think he could either."

"And he can't, can he?"

"He's doing it. He has no choice except *how* to cope with it. Not whether."

"I know."

"Reg—What do you suppose your job is with a man like Antell?"

"Not answering questions?"

"O.K., not answering questions. Then *what?*"

"I know. You've said it before. Listening. Being with him. Trying to understand what's on his mind."

"Maybe there's something about *that* that you feel you can't do."

"Sam, you're asking me to go through it with him."

"You're asking me to let you off the hook. You don't want to suffer."

"Right! I don't!"

"Of course you don't. And neither do I."

Reggie DeBray was in the first stage of training. Clinical training (and "clinical" means "bedside") is designed to let a minister or theological student engage in the work of ministry under supervision. Mostly it's done in hospitals and other places under a Chaplain Supervisor accredited by the Association for Clinical Pastoral Education or one of the other groups that existed until the A.C.P.E. was founded in 1967. I wasn't an accredited supervisor, but a part-time faculty member at Mount Tabor seminary. So students who came to me had to be really hungry for the experience because they wouldn't get any credit for it among clinical-training groups. For long, hard hours of work with me all summer they'd get credit for three hours of course work, and that was all.

But no matter what kind of credit they got, or how much, they were taking the first steps along the road to being pastors. Some of them might wind up as chaplains.

My job: to teach them to examine their work. To examine it clearly, consistently, accurately, with as little personal distortion as possible. To make them able to say that this piece of work was good, that piece bad, that piece passable but improvable. To help them to use that ability to improve their work. To raise tough, hard questions so that they could learn to raise similar questions when a supervisor wasn't around. To help them see that they'd been dependent on teachers and supervisors to tell them what to do, and (by refusing to let them be so dependent on me) to help them to develop themselves as independent practitioners of ministry.

Can you guess, from reading what Reggie DeBray and I said to each other, how he would do as a chaplaincy student?

Does the fact that he failed to call on a dying patient mean that he won't do well as a pastor?

No.

Of course, he did fail his assignment.

But look how little effort it took me to make it possible for Reggie to look at his thoughts, his feelings, his fears. Yes, he was defensive at first, sure that I was going to clobber him. (Later he admitted that he feared I'd wash him out of the program right then.) But what he was able to do—and some students just can't do it—was to say he was afraid, afraid to fail, afraid to tackle tough questions, and mostly, afraid to deal with death (including his own death).

That takes courage.

Courage to feel your fears and not hide them from yourself.

Courage to admit your fears to someone else: the supervisor.

If he could do that, he could learn.

And he did.

You might also be wondering why I didn't *teach* more, tell him more, give him more information about Mr. Antell and patients like him.

As a matter of fact, I sometimes did. And I learned to see that it was a weakness of mine as a supervisor. At that point, I didn't have all the skills I needed—and when I ran out of skills, I gave out information.

Most supervisors learn supervision in the same way I was trying to help students learn to be pastors: by doing the job under the supervision of someone more skilled and advanced. Learning to be a supervisor usually means supervising and taking the process to another supervisor.

That hadn't been my background. I'd been a pastor in a local church for several years and later had gone back to school—at a theological seminary—to earn an advanced degree. Instead of being trained to be a supervisor, I'd been trained to be a scholar and teacher: in fact, to be a seminary professor. I'd gotten a lot of supervision in office counseling, but none in the work of a chaplain. Everything I knew about chaplaincy I'd discovered flying by the seat of my pants.

But there were jobs for chaplains, and not for seminary professors.

What I did, of course, was to take all the teaching techniques in which I'd been trained and carry them right over into supervision. So it was easy to find out *from books* what grief was like, and how it works. And it was all too easy to *tell* the same facts to students. What was hard was to let them find out for themselves, to learn grief by experience, in their guts, rather than in their heads.

What I did with Reginald DeBray was to make it possible and necessary for him to look at himself and how dealing with dying people affected him. It was reasonably good supervision.

I wish I could have done it that way more often.

That same summer, there was a day when Larry Sissman was catching the special calls that came into the office.

I was teaching a class for nursing students when I heard the page come on.

"Chaplain Sissman. Chaplain Lawrence Sissman."

I knew that Audrey, my secretary, was paging him. Something had come up.

Just as the class was over, the page came on again.

"Chaplain Perkins. Chaplain Samuel Perkins."

Dial zero.

THE OPERATOR: Call your office.

AUDREY: They want you up on F-7. That's where I sent Larry.

The ward clerk at the nurses' station on F-7 didn't even speak to me. She just pointed to the door of the doctors' writing room. I could hear an angry voice behind the door.

Inside, Larry Sissman and Charlie Osterman. Charlie was the

AR responsible for F-7. He was chewing Larry out, but when I came in he turned the hose on me.

"I want you to keep your goddam students off the service, Perkins."

"What's up?"

"Never mind what's up. Just get this goddam fuckup off my service!"

Larry's face, already white, went a shade whiter.

Do I walk away? Do I fight it out here? Can I get Osterman slowed down? I'd better try. What will work? Best bet: use my own authority.

"Dr. Osterman, I will not get anybody off any service until I understand what the problem is."

"Can it, Chaplain! I won't have any unprofessional behavior up here."

"Doctor, you are acting unprofessional yourself. I'm just as interested as you are in keeping things straight, up here and everywhere else. *Now, what happened?*"

It worked. He took a deep breath, changed from formal titles to more personal words.

"Aw, dammit, Sam, this man just shook up a patient so bad . . ."

"I *did,* Sam. It's my fault."

"All right. Let's get the details. Go ahead, Charlie."

"Well, he sprung an amputation on a patient before the patient was ready."

"He's right, Sam."

"You're right! I *am* right!"

"See, I stopped by the nurses' desk to find out why they'd called me. And the nurse said that this Mr. Degenhart in 755 was upset. And I asked what about, and she said she didn't know, but she guessed it had something to do with his upcoming amputation. She showed me the chart. He's been getting a lot of stuff for pain . . ."

"And?"

"And so I went in to see him, and he was real depressed, could hardly talk. And I said to him: 'Mr. Degenhart, is it your amputation you're worried about?' And he didn't even know they were going to do one."

"Well, Sam, that's pretty accurate. That's just about what he did. I was passing the door when I heard him say it, and old Degenhart just fainted in the bed: turned white, gulped, fell back onto the pillow."

"How had he been before that, Charlie?"

"Well, he *was* depressed. It was the pain, mostly. It hasn't let up much. But he's kind of a depressed character anyway. We'd had a psychiatric resident up for a consult, and Degenhart wouldn't even talk to him. Having your student up was my idea. I thought if the old guy wouldn't talk to a shrink, he might talk to a preacher. But your guy really fouled it up, talking about the amputation. Now the patient's in there yelling that he won't have his leg off, he'll die first, and all that crap."

"Larry, let's work on it a minute. What was your mistake, as you see it?"

"Talking about the amputation?"

"I don't think so. Not just that, anyhow. There are plenty of cases in which talking about a surgical procedure is just what the patient needs."

"I guess I went in there unprepared."

"Say more about that."

"Well, I just let the nurse tell me stuff, and I didn't pick up that she was just guessing, and I didn't check to see what the patient knew or didn't know."

"O.K."

"And I said too much. Should have let Degenhart lead *me*."

"What do you think, Charlie?" (*Get him to teach instead of scold.*)

"That's right. When you put it that way, I guess I've seen interns do the same thing. More times than I can count."

"Right. Larry, a nurse may be an invaluable source of information. But she may not always know what you need to know, and if you ask her, she may guess."

"So I have to check with the doctor."

"It's a good idea *if* he's around. But you operated in an area where you didn't know the score."

"Don't we have to, sometimes?"

"Sure"—Charlie speaking—"but lay off the guesses and interpretations. You said it right a minute ago: Let the patient lead you."

"Well, where are we?"

"Well, Sam, I think the preacher idea may be a good one, but Sissman here has probably blown it with this patient. Why not send me someone else tomorrow? Nothing personal, kid."

"Sure. I understand."

But I was worried about Larry. It *had* been personal. Charlie Osterman had given him a going over before I even got there, and I wasn't sure what he'd said. And Larry was inept. He had a talent for saying just the wrong thing. In fact, I'd been suspecting that Larry was struggling with a lot of anger toward patients and hadn't been able to come clean with himself about it. I wasn't at all sure what would happen next.

I should have known.

Larry Sissman's supervisory hour the next day. No notes from him. He showed up after a morning supposedly working on Women's Medicine, his pocket patch with the cross on it conspicuously gone.

"Sam, I'd better quit the program."

"Why, Larry?"

"Well, you know how I blew it up on F-7 yesterday? Well, this morning I went to work on Women's Med, and, well, I couldn't talk to anybody."

"Couldn't talk to anybody. I'm not sure I know what that means."

"Well, I'd go into a room and introduce myself, and the . . . well . . . I'd . . . well, I'd . . ." His voice faded away.

"It's pretty painful, isn't it?"

"Oh, God, Sam, I feel like such a fool. I went into five different rooms, and after I said who I was, I just stood there and

didn't say anything. Sam, I can't hack it. I can't stay here. I'll
have to leave. I didn't even do any work you could supervise
me on."

"Larry, stop beating yourself over the head. What do you
think happened this morning? Try to understand it."

"I don't *know!* I guess I didn't want to goof like I goofed
yesterday, and so I just shut up."

We talked about it awhile, not getting much of anywhere.
Larry was too miserable about his failures to be able to examine them. The hour rolled on, with me feeling more and more
that I wasn't able to help him. Finally we were both relieved
when the time was up. At the end, I suggested that we talk
about it in group concerns.

Group concerns is a twice-weekly session when students discuss whatever is important to them, and when they try to deal
with their feelings about the supervisor and each other, to say
nothing of their feelings about doctors, nurses, patients, you
name it.

All four of the students were there, sitting quietly, not talking to each other, when I walked in a little late.

"You're late, Chaplain." (*I had it coming. I'd pointed out
to them that lateness to a group meeting had a meaning. And
in this case the clear meaning was that I too wanted to avoid
what I knew might come.*)

"Yeah. I'm late."

Larry moved right in.

"Look, you guys, I've just about decided to quit."

"What d'ya mean, Larry?"

"Well . . ." And Larry launched into the tale of his mis-
fortunes on F-7 and his painful silences on Women's Medicine.
The way he told the story was a bid for sympathy. He wanted
the other students to realize how miserable and incompetent
he felt. He wasn't prepared for their reaction. Tim Logan spoke
first.

TIM: Gosh, that's too bad. It must feel awful.

DEL: Nonsense. Larry's just bidding for sympathy.

TIM: Aw, I don't think so. Think how awful it'd feel to be tongue-tied with a patient.

DEL: I *know* how awful it'd be. I've *been* tongue-tied with a patient.

REG: Yeah. Me too.

DEL: You think you're the only one with troubles? You're too concerned with yourself, Sissman. I think you just don't like working with patients. You'd rather be sick yourself and getting all the attention.

Larry looked at me with an obvious plea in his eyes to get him out of this situation. I decided to let it go on.

REG: I remember how you always present cases, as if the patient were a nut or a fool or just pretending to be sick. I think Del's right. You just want to be a patient yourself, and you're trying to be a patient in this group.

LARRY: Well, I do want help.

DEL: Sam's already told us that this isn't group therapy in here. We're supposed to look at our work, understand it. Why don't you try to figure out why you couldn't talk?

LARRY: I *have* figured it out.

REG: Well?

And Larry blurted out his revealing answer: "I just figured if they weren't going to talk to me, I wasn't going to talk to them. The hell with a patient who won't cooperate!"

TIM: Whoever said that patients would cooperate? We're there to help them. Not the other way around.

LARRY: You guys are all against me.

TIM: No, we're not.

REG: Yes, we are. We're against self-pity and we're against taking out your problems on the patient. Ever think what it does to a patient to have you stand there mute at the foot of the bed?

LARRY: No. What?

DEL: Well, you ijjit, don't you suppose he might wonder if you're the angel of death, just standing there staring at him?

ME: Larry, what do you think the guys are trying to say to you?

LARRY: That I ought to get out.

REG: No, dummy. We're saying that we don't want to let you run away. We've all had to face stuff too. There was a time when I couldn't even walk into a patient's room. I had to tough it out.

LARRY: You could have quit.

REG: I could have. But I didn't. Perkins wouldn't let me. *I* wouldn't let me. If I didn't deal with it, I'd never be able to face myself. Don't you want to be a pastor?

LARRY: I can preach. I can study the Bible.

DEL: But can you work with people? Real people? Not just faces in the congregation?

LARRY: I don't know. I don't know.

It'd be nice to say that Larry toughed it out for the summer. But he didn't. He stayed on three more weeks and kept walking up to patients, staring at them and not speaking. Finally one day he just didn't show up. I found his pocket patch on my desk.

He made it through Mount Tabor seminary and was ordained. He's pastor of a church somewhere.

And I still wonder if there was a way to reach him.

Many theological schools are requiring clinical pastoral education as a part of ministerial training. It's almost the only place in theological education where a man can look (*must* look) at the way he works with people. Clinical training is still not a part of the training of most ministers.

It *is* required by most hospitals now as a necessary condition of working in the hospital as a chaplain. I wish it were universally required.

But I'm prejudiced.

X

BEHIND THE STAIRS

CHAPLAIN TO WHOM?

It's more of a question than you might think.

In some hospitals the chaplain is chaplain just to the patients. But at MUH the Hospital Administrator was careful to say that I was to be the chaplain to the *hospital*. The whole hospital was to be my parish: patients, staff, employees.

Lots of the work was just a matter of responding to the little things that cropped up here and there. Like my daily call on Naida Littleton, the Director of Admissions. Just five minutes.

Naida had been to hotel school at Cornell. The administration was wise to pick someone with her background, because a hospital is a hotel. I won't bore you with word games, but in fact the word "hospital" and the word "hotel" have the same roots.

"G'morning, Naida. How's it going?"

"As usual, Chaplain. We'll never fit 'em all in."

"Maybe I should've asked how bad it is."

"Yeah. It's always bad, just a question of how bad it is."

"Is it tough all over?"

"Better here than in most places. Why, at Saint Cosmas' they have patients bedded down in the hospital corridors. I'd shut down before I did that."

"Naida, what's your toughest problem?"

"Race."

"Race?"

"Race. Y'didn't know that, didya?"

"I still don't understand it."

"Well, y'see, there's no race problem in the private rooms. Anybody with the money to pay for it can get a bed there, *if* I've got a single room. But the minute I put a black person in semiprivate or a ward, I've got to worry about what the other patients will say. Some of them want out immediately.

"But it's even worse in the house services. Not medicine, for some reason. But, you know, every room in the house services is a four-bed room. If I put a black person in a four-bed room on surgery, I've got to empty the room, or else put nothing but blacks in it. We have to have black rooms and white rooms. And you know what's the worst?"

"No."

"OB-GYN. We just plain can't accept blacks in that service at all. The doctors, the patients, the families—they all get up in arms if I put a black lady in a room with white women. And they're worse about it there than anywhere else."

"Why?"

"Ask the psychiatrists. Seriously, I do think it's got something to do with sex. OB-GYN is a sexy service—at least in the sense that patients there are always dealing with something sexual. Maybe it bothers white women to see a black father walk in to visit his woman."

"His woman?"

"You mean why don't I say his *wife?* Well, I guess I'm prejudiced too. Actually, of course, we get marrieds and unmarrieds. I don't ask."

"What do *you* do about it, Naida?"

"Ha! I keep annoying the doctors. I think (even if I *am* prejudiced) that every bed in the hospital has to be open to anybody. The Federal Government is going to say that soon anyway, if it hasn't already. In my book it's a practical issue. But I guess for you it's a moral issue."

"I think it's probably both."

"Well, I suppose so. It sure creates problems for me."

"Naida, it must cost the hospital a lot of money to have 'black' rooms and 'white' rooms."

"Of course it does. I don't know how much."

"Maybe that's a way to attack the problem. Have you ever added up what it does to our costs to keep things that way? No, you just said you haven't. Why not add it up and present it to the Director's Office? They're always interested in keeping costs down."

"I think I will. I bet we could save a lot. And, you know, it *is* a moral issue. People are people, and we ought to treat them as people."

A telephone call from Dr. Abbott, the professor of anatomy in the medical school.

"Chaplain Perkins, this is Geoffrey Abbott. I have a strange request to make of you."

"Yes?"

"In three weeks we'll be through with anatomical dissection. Would it be appropriate for you to say the burial service for the cadavers? I know it's a little odd, but it seems right to me."

"A private burial service?"

"I think not. I'd really like to have you do it in class, with the medical students present. Would there be any complications? Are you free to do that sort of thing?"

"Yes, I'm free to do what seems appropriate to me."

"Are there any problems?"

"Only this: Why with the medical students present? I'm not against that, but I do wonder what you have in mind."

"I think medical students should be reverent. Even if they are not religious in the traditional Jewish or Christian sense, they should be reverent toward those cadavers."

"Then perhaps what would be appropriate would be a service of thanksgiving."

"That would be excellent."

And so, three weeks later, in a long, drab room smelling of formalin, among forty men of religious and nonreligious convictions, with ten draped forms on the white enamel tables, the words of burial:

". . . and though this body be destroyed, yet shall I see God: whom I shall see for myself, and mine eyes shall behold, and not as a stranger . . .

". . . grant to us who are still in our pilgrimage, and who walk as yet by faith, that having served thee with constancy on earth . . .

". . . we yield unto thee most high praise and hearty thanks for those from whom we have been privileged to learn. And, as they in dying gave us this last gift, may we give to our patients that same measure of devotion and care . . .

". . . unto Almighty God we commend our brothers and sisters departed, and we commit their bodies to the fire, grateful that in their deaths there is life for others. Amen."

Afterward.

"Chaplain, I'm an atheist, and I guess I don't believe that God stuff you were talking about."

"Not everyone does."

"But I guess I'm not a materialist. And what I do believe is that I really should be grateful even to these cadavers for the opportunity to learn. For that part, I thank you."

"You're very welcome."

"This anatomy stuff has been pretty easy. First time I'd seen dead bodies. Some of it was hard, though."

"What part was hardest, Mr. Freund?"

"The hands."

"Ever figure out why?"

"No. Maybe, though, it's because even these preserved hands have calluses and stuff that make them look pretty real."

"More human than other parts of the body?"

"Yeah. I think my cadaver must've been a carpenter."

Later, I heard that some doctors at Tulane had written about the emotional problems of medical students. They said the same thing: that dissecting hands was one of the toughest parts of anatomy.

I see that I've written about the funeral for the cadavers as though it had been simply a matter of "Will you?" "Yes." and the deed was done. From the outside, I guess that's how it would have looked to anyone. But it's not really the way it was.

That "burial service" cost me as much mental agony as anything I ever did as a chaplain.

Not because it was a funeral: I'd often done that.

Not because it was connected with cadavers and dissection: I'd already dealt with death and dead bodies in a number of ways.

I think what bothered me most was Dr. Abbott's assumption that a ritual was needed. A ritual that perhaps only he could appreciate. Maybe it was his assumption that chaplains were in hospitals for the purpose of maintaining pious rituals, or his thought that the flesh can't be disposed of without ceremony.

Maybe he was right.

I can imagine that some families might be comforted to know that Uncle Joe, who had donated his body to medical research, was finally buried (or, in this case, cremated) with proper last rites.

And it's not a bad idea to be reverent or grateful about the gift of knowledge.

And perhaps it's all right to ask a chaplain, who in some way "represents religion" in the hospital, to represent the gratitude and reverence of people in a service like this one.

But it bothered me. It felt like a ritual without much meaning. It didn't represent the thoughts and feelings of the medical students. The cadavers were long since dead, and those who loved them as people had long since said the good-bys that had meaning. So, in part, this service felt pagan to me.

Pagan?

Yes, because ritual for ritual's sake is always pagan. If it is not really a part of living people's response to a living God, it's just a quick nod in the direction of an idol.

Of course, a lot of our practice of religion is pagan, in that sense. A "Hail Mary" said with the lips but not the heart, the Lord's Prayer muttered from memory without meaning, the Seder meal observed because Grandpa would be upset if we didn't—these are pagan rather than really Christian or really Jewish.

Still, I participated. In fact, I led the service. It might be, for a few, a way of expressing their real gratitude. It might be a means for some to recollect their dependence on others, or on an Other.

What is a constructive compromise? Did I find one here?

And what about this one?

Mark Partin, rabbi of the conservative congregation in town, stuck his head in my office door.

"Sam."

"Yo, Mark."

"Got time to come to a 'briss'?"

"Sure do."

So down the hall we went. I thought how funny it is to have a briss (the ancient Jewish ritual of circumcision) in a modern hospital. How would they handle it? Would they really have a "mohel"? (The religious functionary whose job it is to circumcise.)

They had a mohel. It was Bernie Glassman, one of MUH's best surgeons. He could satisfy the ritual requirements and at the same time maintain hospital sterility standards.

So the squalling Blitzstein boy was circumcised, and the grandfathers toasted one another with love and joy in their eyes. Bernie took a glass of wine too and went home.

Another ritual? No different from the funeral?

I think I see a difference.

Here were people celebrating the joy of life before God as they felt it and experienced it right now. Right at that moment their feelings were expressed in a lively way within their own tradition. I was pleased to be a guest.

They brought the baby over for me to see—not to bless, for I was not of their tradition. I wanted to speak to him. I looked at the glowing father. What was there to say?

"Hello, ben b'rith" (son of the covenant).

He went on squalling. But isn't that a baby's business?

How can I tell you about the routine and the drudgery?

Some days were made up of nothing else.

One set of notes for a particular day says only: forty calls today. Forty times talking with a patient. Forty times when something maybe happened, or nothing did. Just answering the phone, answering the page, walking the halls, no particular incidents, no struggles; a routine of lives beginning, lives being prolonged, lives being saved, lives ending.

I borrowed a pedometer for a few days and clocked myself along the halls. Seven miles, ten miles, and once, fourteen miles in a day.

The Hospital Administrator got worried about what I should wear.

Clothes tell you what status a person has.

Medical students wear street clothes and a short white jacket.

Interns wear a white shirt and white pants—no coat.

Residents wear a white jacket and white pants.

Chief residents in a service wear a white shirt, black tie, white jacket, and white pants.

The upper echelons—attending physicians, teaching staff, physicians beyond their training years—wear their street clothes, but put on a long white lab coat.

In some hospitals—but not MUH—you'd better look at that clothing carefully because it tells you who gets on the elevator first, and you get chewed out if you get on the elevator before somebody who outranks you. At MUH that was considered Mickey Mouse.

What does the chaplain wear?

I wore my street clothes and had a cross emblem that hung out of my handkerchief pocket. My tradition didn't call for a clerical collar, though I wore one for services of worship.

The administrator thought that I should dress more appropriately to my rank. What rank? Well, he said, I should wear a long white lab coat.

He quoted the old adage about hospitals: "Wear a long white coat and you can go anywhere. Have a stethoscope sticking out of the side pocket and you can do anything."

At lunch, I chuckled over it all with a sociologist friend, an enemy of organized religion.

"I've got it all figured out," said Jerry.

"What've you got all figured out?"

"Didn't you say you had to pray over the dedication of the new wing?"

"Yeah."

"Well, look—wear your clerical collar *and* a long white lab coat. You'll symbolize religion and medicine at the same time. You can do the whole damn prayer by nonverbal communication!"

I reported the conversation to the Hospital Administrator as a good joke.

I should've known better.

He thought it was a good idea.

XI
PATIENTHOOD

THE TWO-HUNDRED-SEAT CLASSROOM was full of teen-age girls, going through a training program so that they'd be useful volunteers—the kind known as "candy stripers." Jayne Martin, the Volunteer Services Director, had asked me to give one of the training lectures.

"Sam," said Jayne, "I'm going to ask you to talk to them about something no doctor ever understands."

"What's that?" I asked, sure that she meant something like "Religion in the Hospital."

"How It Feels to Be a Patient."

Now, as I was about to start my lecture, I had a mental flashback. In my imagination, I was once again standing at the bedside of Hank Henrici, Chief of the Hematology Service. Hank, a determined if clumsy athlete, had broken his leg playing touch football with his seven sons.

"Boy, Chaplain, this is some lesson!"

"Never to play touch football at the age of forty-eight?"

"No, you dirty dog!" said Hank with a grin. "It's a lesson in patienthood. You've heard the old saw that doctors make lousy patients? Well, I'm learning why."

"What do you think you're learning, Hank?"

"Well, you know I'm in the Naval Reserve? How do you think it would feel to go to bed as captain of your ship and wake up the next morning as a lousy able-bodied seaman?"

"So it feels like a real loss of rank, eh?"

"And how! Y'know, Sam, we *say* that hospitals are dedicated to the welfare of the patient . . ."

"D'you think we don't really mean it?"

"Oh, we mean it all right. But we make the patient pay a hell of a price. He's got to acknowledge that he's at the bottom of the totem pole. He must admit that everybody outranks him, right down to the aide who moves bedpans. He has to give up his right to ask questions such as: What's that medicine for? He has to make himself over into a totally passive object— something for other people to do things to."

"Hey, that really gripes you, doesn't it?"

"Yeah. And you know what gripes me most of all? It's that I do the same thing. I don't *want* patients asking me a lot of questions about 6-mercaptopurine. [A drug used in the treatment of serious blood diseases.] I want them to take their medicine quietly and to believe that the doctor knows best. And I'll bet that when I get out of here I'll forget all I've learned and go right on riding roughshod over the feelings of patients."

"Hank, could that be changed? Does it have to happen that way?"

"Well, I don't really know, Sam. They never even try to teach us in med school how it feels to be a patient. In fact, if we knew too much about that, we might even be poorer doctors."

"How's that?"

"Well, maybe I can't *afford* to feel the fear that clutches at some patient's throat when the word 'leukemia' is floating around."

"You can't afford to lose your cold, scientific outlook, is that it?"

"Exactly. But right now I'm feeling all the things you lose when you become a patient. That's what it means to be a patient: loss."

Now all of that conversation came back. And I said to the prospective candy stripers:

To be a patient means losing a lot. What do you lose when you're a patient?

—You lose space. When you're well, your world consists of houses, fields, streets, open spaces, closed spaces—all kinds of space. As a patient, your world is ten feet by ten feet if you're lucky. It may be even smaller. Your world really shrinks.

—You lose mobility. As you get better—*if* you get better—they may let you move around, up and down the hall. For some patients, being allowed to go to the john on their own is a privilege they look forward to for weeks.

—You lose control over who invades your space. At home, you don't have to let anybody in. Nobody. Unless he has a search warrant. When you're a patient, dozens of people suddenly have the right to come right up to you and touch you, and there's nothing you can do about it. Most of them don't even say "excuse me."

—You lose control over time. You do things when other people want you to, not when you want to. Have you heard the old bitter joke about being awakened at midnight to take a sleeping pill? It is not a joke. It happens in this hospital.

Our patients who are well acquainted with the Bible often remind me of a passage in which Jesus says to Peter: "when you were young you fastened your belt about you and walked where you chose; but when you are old you will stretch out your arms, and a stranger will bind you fast, and carry you where you have no wish to go." (John 21:18, NEB.) Jesus wasn't really talking about what it feels like to be a patient, but to many patients the words ring true.

—You lose control over what's done to your body. For most healthy people, their skin is a kind of barrier; nobody can get inside your skin unless you want them to. But being a patient means that people get inside your skin—with tubes, needles, liquids, and probes.

—You lose contact, and maybe that's the worst of all. You can't go to people; they have to come to you. And sometimes they don't come.

What does that add up to?

It adds up to words like this:

—lonely

—isolated

—shut in

—caged

—helpless

That in turn adds up to words like:

—angry

—suspicious

—irritable

—demanding.

I guess I said some other things to the candy stripers, but that's what I really wanted to get said.

Detective tale.

At lunch one day with the interns and the AR from one of the Men's Medicine sections, I heard them puzzling over a patient.

". . . but there's nothing to account for it. He doesn't even have that kind of illness."

"Well, then, dammit, he's got more than one illness. *Something* has to account for it."

"Excuse me, Chaplain. Hey, you guys talking about Doc Holliday?"

"Yeah."

"Who's Doc Holliday?"

"Well, Chaplain, it's the damndest thing you ever saw. His name isn't really Holliday, but he is a doctor. An old-timer from out in the country, in general practice for God knows how long."

"Something odd going on with him?"

"Yeah. He's got a case of emphysema—not too bad yet. But there's something else wrong, and we can't figure it out. To be blunt about it, he shits the bed."

"I take it you can't figure out his loss of bowel control?"

"Right!"

"What does he say about it?"

"Not a thing. Just looks at you with those funny blue eyes of his and apologizes. I could swear he's laughing."

"It might be possible that he really is laughing, huh?"

"Well, Chaplain, it might be, but why? Hey, why don't you go see him? He's an interesting old coot."

He *was* interesting. I stopped by to see him, and before I knew it, I'd spent almost an hour just chatting casually with him. The subject of his bowels never came up. But the old man seemed so alert and lively that I couldn't believe in his loss of control.

I stopped one of the interns, Bill Muskie, in the hall.

"Bill, about Doctor Treadwell . . ."

"Who?"

"Doc Holliday."

"Oh . . . Something I can help you with?"

"Well, this business of his losing bowel control. Can you tell me more about it?"

"Nothing much. Just that it happens every day."

"When every day?"

"About seven thirty in the evening."

"You mean it? Same time every day?"

"Just about. Why?"

"I've got an idea. You on tonight?"

"Yep."

"Meet me outside Doc Holliday's room about four thirty?"

"I can. But why?"

"Well, just you play Dr. Watson and let me be Sherlock Holmes for two more hours."

At four thirty, Muskie and I met and went to look for Arthur Moore, the aide.

"Arthur, can we talk to you a minute."

"Sure."

"You know about Dr. Treadwell and his bowel problem?"

"You mean how he shits the bed? Yeah, I know, but I ain't never taken care of him."

"Why not?"

"I always been on break when it happens."

"Arthur, would you be willing to give up your break this evening? It's for a good cause."

"Well, I guess so."

So Arthur Moore did not go on break that Wednesday evening. And Dr. Treadwell did not lose bowel control.

The next day Bill Muskie and I went to see Doc Holliday.

"Dr. Treadwell."

"Well, Chaplain, looks like a formal call. And you've got Dr. Muskie with you!"

"We have a couple of questions to ask you."

"Fire away!"

"What's the name of the night charge nurse on this section?"

"Miss Strunk." His lips were compressed, his eyes wary.

"You don't like her, do you?"

"Like her! If that nurse worked for me, she'd last less than a day. She sticks needles into people just to see them squirm, pushes them around. Nobody who hates people that much should be allowed to be a nurse!"

And Muskie couldn't wait. He dove in.

"And that's why you lose bowel control, isn't it?"

"I don't know what you mean, Doctor."

"Oh, yes, you do, *Doctor*. You wait until Arthur goes on break, so he won't have to clean it up, because you like Arthur. The minute he's off the floor, you just let it rip, don't you?" Because you know that Arabella Strunk is going to have to clean it up. There's not a damn thing wrong with your colon!"

"Well, Doctor, I'll tell you . . . you're absolutely right. There isn't much I can do to that old bitch of a nurse who's a disgrace to her calling—so I did what I could. Now that you have it figured out, I'll have to stop it. But I'll tell you something: it was worth it."

Some of the house staff suggested that all of this was evidence that Dr. Treadwell had seriously regressed psychologically. They wanted psychiatric consultation, commitment to the state hospital, all sorts of controls.

But Dr. Treadwell never lost control again. And he had support from many house doctors. They, too, thought that Arabella Strunk had it coming. Being a patient means that there's little you can do about a mean nurse. If you complain, there are dozens of little ways she can pay you back. In fact, all she has to do is to be slow in answering when you push the button. Many times that's punishment enough. She has power, and you have none. There aren't many ways you can deal with it.

Dr. Treadwell found a way.

Being a patient often means being confused about what you see and hear, sure only that dangerous, difficult, and even fatal things await you.

The late Ogden Nash, whose poetry was usually so amusing, wrote a serious poem that *The New Yorker* printed just as I was leaving MUH. I clipped it out and kept it.

NOTES FOR THE CHART IN 306

The bubbles soar and die in the sterile bottle
Hanging upside down on the bedside lamppost.
Food and drink
Seep quietly through the needle strapped to the hand.
The arm welcomes the sting of mosquito hypodermic—
Conveyor of morphia, the comforter.
Here's drowsiness, here's lassitude, here's nothingness,
Sedation *in excelsis.*
The clouded mind would stray into oblivion
But for the grackle-squawk of the box in the hall,
The insistent call for a faceless goblin horde
Of sorcerers, vivisectionists, body-snatchers.
Dr. Polyp is summoned,
Dr. Gobbo and Dr. Prodigy,
Dr. Tortoise, Dr. Sawdust, and Dr. Mary Poppins,
La belle dame sans merci.
Now it's Dr. Bandarlog and Dr. Bacteria,
And last of all, the terrifying one,
Dodger Thomas.
And there is no lock on the door.

On the third day, the goblins are driven off
To the operating room beneath the hill.
Dr. Vandeleur routs gibbering Bandarlog,
Bacteria flees before swarthy Dr. Bagderian.
Sawdust and Polyp yield to Saunders and Pollitt,
And it's Porter instead of Tortoise who knocks at the door.
He will test the blood, not drain it.
The eerie impostors are gone, all gone but one—
Dodger Thomas.
I know he is lurking somewhere in a shadow.
Dodger Thomas.
I've never met him, but old friends have.
I know his habit:
He enters without knocking.

"Mr. Ravitch, I'm Chaplain Perkins." (*Surgery tomorrow for him.*)

"I'm glad you came."

"They seem to have you hooked up to a good many tubes here."

"Isn't that the truth? They're trying to get me well enough to operate on me."

"Yes, and I hear they've succeeded."

"No kidding? They're going to operate?"

"Yes. I thought you already knew." (*A flash of anger. Surgery tomorrow morning and he hadn't even known it. Has he had a chance to call his wife a hundred and fifty miles away?*)

"No. I didn't know. Is it tomorrow?"

"Yes, it is."

"Gee, Chaplain, could you call Yvonne and tell her for me?"

"I'd be glad to."

"Chaplain, I know you're not a doctor, but maybe you could tell me . . . What is the operation I'm going to have?"

Anger again.

"Hasn't the doctor told you?"

"Well, yes, he has, as a matter of fact, but I don't understand it. I thought maybe you could help me. It's a mastic section, or something like that."

You don't tell him. You get a doctor. I went out and found Ralph Squair, brought him into the room.

"Dr. Squair, Mr. Ravitch here was asking about his surgery, and I wondered if you could give us a few minutes."

"Sure. Now, Mr. Ravitch, what we're going to do tomorrow is a gastric resection. O.K.?"

Mr. Ravitch smiled weakly.

"Doctor, I wonder if Mr. Ravitch knows what a gastric resection is?"

"Oh. Well, what it really means is that we're going to remove a portion of your stomach, Mr. Ravitch."

"How will I digest food?"

"What do you mean?"

"Well, without a stomach and all."

"Sam, would you hand me that piece of rubber tubing? Thanks. Now, Mr. Ravitch, what we'll do, you see, is to remove a piece of your stomach. Your stomach is like a large tube, and we'll take out a whole section (and with a pocketknife Dr. Squair did just that to the rubber tubing) and then take the two parts that are left open and join them to each other—like this. Sew them up, and you'll be eating as good as new in a few days. O.K.?"

"Thank you very much, Doctor. That helps."

"Very welcome." And Ralph Squair left the room.

"Chaplain."

"Yes, Mr. Ravitch."

"Thanks. I understand better, and now I'm not so scared. Yvonne, she wouldn't want the doctor to show her, but me, I do. But it's a big operation, don't you think?"

"Still seems pretty big to you?"

"Well, you know, I can't move, and I can't even go to the bathroom for myself. A man lies here and thinks, and things get bigger and bigger. If your body isn't going, your mind imagines up all kinds of things. You know?"

"Particularly when you can't do much for yourself . . ."

"All I can do is think. Sometimes thinking gets out of control."

"Like your mind can't stop." (*Still trying to help him say all he needs to say.*)

"Your believing changes too."

"How is that, Mr. Ravitch?" (*I really wasn't expecting it.*)

"You wonder. Does God care? Is he maybe just forgetting you, like the doctors and nurses do sometimes? I push the bell, I can't get a nurse. Maybe I can't get God either. Is that bad, thinking that way?"

(*Temptation: Tell him it's bad theology to think of God as something at the other end of a push button. Supervisory answer: Why is he saying that? What's cooking for him?*)

"Mr. Ravitch, I guess it's pretty frightening to think you can't get through to God—or to anyone else who might help."

"Yessir, it is. But *you* came."

Sometimes you pull together the threads of a conversation in a prayer, so that the patient's fears and feelings are offered to God. That's what I did this afternoon.

"Lord, please hear how good and how bad we feel. We thank you for the surgeons who are going to help Mr. Ravitch tomorrow. We are grateful for their skill. We thank you for the nurses, and are grateful for their care. But hear too, Lord, the feeling that an operation is a big and frightening thing to have happen. Help Mr. Ravitch to feel calm and secure. Help him to trust in you and in the people to whom you gave these abilities to heal. For the past few days Mr. Ravitch has been lying very still. He knows that it was important, but he wants to move. Help him to put up with lying still just a little longer. For Jesus' sake. Amen."

"Thank you, Chaplain."

"You're welcome."

"I guess the Lord knew all along how it was, but I needed to have it said."

It's eleven thirty. The shifts have changed. By midnight all the nurses will be caught up with what's going on on their services. Patients are NPO'd for surgery the next morning.

I've been in the Emergency Room. There was a neighborhood brawl, and one man was shot. I sat with his wife and children until Dr. Menges came out to say that he would live. What Menges didn't tell them was that he would never walk again. The shot severed his spinal cord. He left that for someone on Men's Surgery to do, tomorrow or the next day.

But Menges told me.

Walking up to Men's Surgery with the family, I feel dishonest. I know something they don't know, and I am giving them reassurance: half true, half lie.

Once they're sure he's settled for the night, they're willing to go home. I write a little note to the AR for the service, warning him that the family does not know the extent of Mr. Sugrue's condition. I also tell him that I have a working relationship with the family and will be available in the morning to talk with him or them.

On the Men's Surgery hall, the lights are dimmed for the night, except for the bright spot at the nurses' station. Around the corner in Peds, the halls are brightly lighted.

The page comes on.

"Dr. Toffler. Dr. Arthur Toffler."

There is no Arthur Toffler on the staff. It is the code for a postmortem examination. Someone has died. A post permission has been signed. The pathologists are being roused from sleep, to gather in silence around an enameled table. The chief pathologist insists on a silence that borders on reverence. Only the chapel is quieter.

I walk past the admission desk, where Kay Sturgeon is admitting a mother-to-be.

I stop at the door to chat briefly with Carl Teague, who will deliver the mother. He was leaving, but is coming back in.

The page.

"Dr. Terman. Dr. Edgar Terman."

The Emergency Room.

I guess I'm not going home yet, either.

p. 91